Making a Difference:
One Man's Journey

By: Herb Sandmire M.D.

TO Bill Dittman, my med-
school classmate, with my
best wishes.

Herb Sandmire

First published by Dog Ear Publishing
4010 W. 86th Street, Ste H
Indianapolis, IN 46268
www.dogearpublishing.net

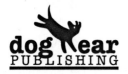

ISBN: 978-145750-423-5

This book is printed on acid-free paper.

Printed in the United States of America

Acknowledgements

With deep gratitude, I acknowledge the proofing and editorial assistance of David Sandmire.

I also acknowledge my wife of 59 years, Crystal, for the foresight she had more than 60 years ago of keeping interesting things preserved in 46 scrapbooks. It borders on the bizarre that seemingly she knew I would be publishing an autobiography some 60 years later in 2011 and she would be able to provide me with more information than I could possibly use. Without that foresight, this book could not have been written. Furthermore, I acknowledge her superb computer skills, all of which she taught herself. Those skills have been absolutely necessary in the process of putting this book together.

Contents

Preface

*If I have seen a little further, it is by standing
on the shoulders of Giants.*

—Isaac Newton,
in a letter to his intellectual rival, Robert Hooke, February 5, 1676.

FOR THE PAST 15 years, my wife and children have urged me to write about my life and experiences. Until recently, I resisted this suggestion, thinking that no one would be interested in my memoirs. However, my retirement "in phases" has given me more time to reflect on what I have seen and done in my 82 years – time to "come up for air," so to speak. So in August of 2010, I put pen to paper and began writing.

I am blessed to live in a country where a dirt-poor kid from a tenant farming family in Wisconsin can seize opportunities presented to achieve a top-notch education and become a successful physician. In my wildest childhood dreams, I wouldn't have imagined any of this would happen, nor would my parents, who did not know of my intentions to pursue medical school until I received my acceptance letter from the University of Wisconsin (UW) Medical School's Dean William S. Middleton.

As is often the case in life, both motivation and serendipity shaped my personal and professional path. A case of mistaken identity during a blind-date in college led me to Crystal Ainsworth, the woman who would become my wife and closest companion for the next 60 years, with whom I would have five children, ten grandchildren, and would travel to five continents. Together, "Sweetie" and I saw Bart Starr cross the goal line in the legendary Ice Bowl and watched the smoke rise over the Pentagon while in Washington, D.C. during the 9-11 attacks. Our highest highs and lowest lows were spent together, and even if I could, I would not have changed any of it.

After my college chemistry instructor, in hushed tones, told me that another student was looking over my shoulder for correct answers during an exam, I summoned the nerve to switch majors from Agriculture Education to Chemistry – a serendipitous event that placed me into a class with all Pre-med students and ultimately changed my life forever. In another scene of pure happenstance, when the three trained obstetricians at the 5001st USAF Hospital in Fairbanks, Alaska were discharged following the Korean War, I, as a general medical officer, was given a crash course in forceps and cesarean deliveries. Within six months, at 25 years of age, I became the chief of an obstetric service delivering 125 babies a month. This led to a residency in obstetrics and gynecology at the University of Iowa and a career in obstetrics with just under 11,000 babies delivered and over 40 scientific publications during the next six decades.

The changes in medicine over the past 60 years have been truly astounding. When I walked through the doors of UW Medical School for the first time in 1949, we didn't even know the structure of DNA. Sixty years later, the entire human genome has been mapped. I have had the good fortune to witness this unfolding of modern medicine from the vantage point of obstetrics and gynecology, and I have tried, in my small way, to contribute to this medical revolution. As the costs of technological medicine sky-rocketed, I worked to hold costs down by founding Wisconsin's first, non-hospital-affiliated, outpatient Surgical Center, demonstrating the practicality of uterine curettage as an office procedure, and delivering health care to patients at Green Bay's Free Clinic. My published work helped the medical community establish more cost-effective practices for the use of Pap smears and the screening for sexually transmitted diseases and generated support for the notion of cost savings inherent in the training of medical assistants for an expanded role in health care.

As Isaac Newton recognized three centuries ago, none of our thinking arises in isolation. We are shaped by those who came before us. My own circumstances would not have been possible without the professors and clinicians who guided my development in the formative years.

This realization has driven my own efforts to share my expertise with others as the preceptor in charge of fourth year UW medical student training from 1966 to 1986, the founding medical director of the Green Bay Obstetric Rotation from 1980 to 2010, and the founding medical director of the Green Bay Mini-fellowship program established in 1985. I've been honored with the opportunity, as an emeritus clinical faculty member in UW's Departments of Family Medicine and Obstetrics and Gynecology, to help train more than 700 U.S. physicians and have served as a tutor for countless others who were judged by Medical Examining Boards to need remedial work.

Most professions are fraught with ethical questions, and obstetrics and gynecology is no exception. Holding firm to one's convictions is, I believe, as important as one's technical knowledge in a field. My dedication to preserving women's reproductive rights has been unwavering. Our 1971 founding of Green Bay's Planned Parenthood Clinic provided young women with much-needed privacy and guidance in matters of contraception and pregnancy. The historic 1973 *Row v. Wade* U.S. Supreme Court ruling legalizing abortion has spawned many lawsuits in the years since – one of the earliest was ours, *Doe v. Bellin Memorial Hospital*, in which a Green Bay hospital denied the right of my patient to receive an abortion (a case that worked its way up to the U.S. Supreme Court). Our medical clinic's continued provision of women's reproductive services has not come without protest – our offices have been picketed regularly for the past 37 years (and even my home, on occasion).

Nonetheless, through all of the tumult and uncertainty inherent in "taking a stand," it has been gratifying to realize that not everyone out there is a detractor. I've been humbled to receive, over the years, nineteen teaching and professional awards from state, national, and international organizations, the most recent being the Distinguished Service Award from the 50,000-member American College of Obstetricians and Gynecologists and my selection as an Honorary Member of the French National College of Gynecologists and Obstetricians – the latter of which I received during a gourmet banquet dinner in the Eiffel Tower with Sweetie, my daughters, my daughters-in-law, and my granddaughter by my side. Not bad for a dirt-poor farm boy from Wisconsin who's just happy to be alive.

CHAPTER 1

The early years

I WAS BORN in Richland Center, Wisconsin on the ninth of April, 1929, the seventh child of Carl Glen and Lois Bernadine Sandmire. Two more children (Janet Bernadine and Lyle LaVaughn) followed my birth. My father was a tenant farmer, meaning we rented the farm and were required to pay one half of the farm profit to the owner.

My first ten to eleven years of life was during the Great Depression of the 1930s. Despite this, we raised our own food (vegetables, beef, pork and chickens), were never, in my memory, hungry, nor did we lack any other essential needs including clothing, some of which was made by my mother. In fact, my parents bought a new Terraplane Hudson motor car during the extremely hot, 1936 summer and took a trip to Yellowstone National Park.

Despite our modest upbringings, my brothers, sisters, and I made our way in the world. By 1934, Cardell, the oldest of us, finished high school and went off to Normal School for one year as preparation for receiving a teacher's certificate. Coming home for the weekends, she would resume "bossing me around," whereupon I'd inform her "you do not live here anymore!" The truth was, none of us lived there much longer since tenant farm work required us to move frequently.

On March 1st, 1941, to be closer to the University of Wisconsin at Madison, our family moved to Cottage Grove. I, at age eleven, was sent a week ahead of the rest of the family to ascertain which of the 40 cows currently needed to be milked. Cottage Grove, at that time, was a small village of 309 people about eight miles east of Madison. The farm we rented was right in the center of the village, directly across the street from the Post Office. Therefore, we enjoyed both the farm and "city life" from which I have many fond memories. Our farming life,

1

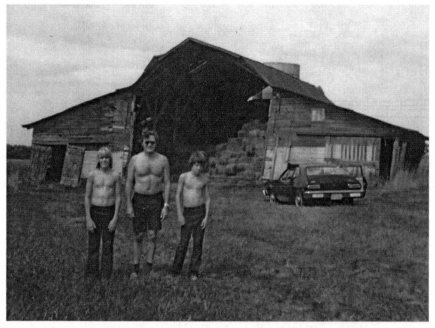

Visiting my birth farm with my two youngest sons (1975)

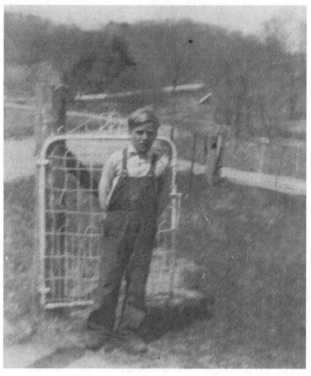

At the front of our one room school at eight years of age. (Spring 1937)

especially its efficiency, in Cottage Grove was vastly improved over Richland County by the purchase of a small Allis Chalmers tractor to assist our team of horses in the fieldwork. The Clark farm, which we rented, was large at 240 acres, and the tractor was small, necessitating round-the-clock usage. From age 11 through 15, I was one of the tractor operators, generally taking the evening shift, and was often accompanied by one of my girl friends. For farm life, you can't beat that!

Looking back on it, life on the farm was not easy but did not seem too bad. It involved getting up at 5:30 am, helping to milk by hand, 40 cows, having breakfast and heading off to school. The milking procedure was repeated each evening, 365 days a year (366 in a leap year!).

At age 14, I "borrowed" my older brother Cameron's motorcycle, lost control going over the railroad tracks, and cut open the inside of my left knee. I can, 68 years later, still smell the open drop ether that the nurse administered while the physician placed 31 stitches to bring the wound edges together.

Perhaps I should digress at this point and describe my unscholarly record in grades seven, eight, nine and ten at the Cottage Grove school and eleven and twelve at Madison East High School. Incidentally, I was called Foster – my middle name – throughout high school after which I used my first name, which is Herbert. This may have been my not too subtle attempt to erase my high school academic record from the books. At any rate, I will identify the low point of all my report cards for one grading period in ninth grade:

> *English C-, Business Practice C-, Science F and Citizenship F. Times tardy 4 and absent 7 days.*

When my mother asked how I could explain such a report card containing two C-s and two Fs, I responded, "I guess I concentrated too much on two subjects!" Other report cards outlining my lack of scholarly production during junior high at Cottage Grove included, for one reporting period:

Foster Sandmire   3rd Period
Is doing excellent work in   ____none_____
Is working to capacity in   _____none_____
Is doing good work in   _____Science_____
Is in need of improvement in   all subjects except science
Especially commendable characteristics :   cheerfulness
Suggestions for improvement: Study every day. Makes good start and

then slackens in his work – has 70 average in English so far this semester.
Teacher's comment: *He has applied himself a little more lately, but can do*
even better in science. He works like a trooper for a couple of weeks and
then takes it easy for a while. Recent English project was not acceptable.
Only fair in Music workbook.

My mother's response to the teacher read: *"Will see you soon concerning the English. I can't understand his explanations of the test given in
English."*

The English project assignment was to provide a stage that could
be used for a Shakespearean play. I picked up an empty box on the way
to school and indicated to the teacher that, without other "props," it
would accentuate the natural talents of the actors and actresses. Apparently, the teacher did not share my enthusiasm for the idea.

Another report card went like this:

Foster Sandmire 1ˢᵗ Period
Is doing good work in _____*English, Science*_____
Is in need of improvement __*Citizenship, Business Practice*__
Especially commendable characteristics __*Always ready to help in school,*
*better attitude, a gentleman.*__ (Apparently, I excelled in deportment –
with excellent behavioral characteristics)
More homework – one subject prepared thoroughly each night
*Foster is fully capable of doing better work. I think he did better work last
year; however, he has shown improvement recently.*
Use care in workbook. Could show more interest in singing.

My main failing at the junior high level at Cottage Grove, as
reported by the teachers, was the lack of application – *"he could do better."* Each time we had our IQ test and the findings of my performance
returned to the school, I was prepared for the refrain, *"Foster can do better."* The consensus of the teachers seemed to be that *"Foster was a very
nice gentleman, filled with cheerfulness, highly considerate of others but with
limited cognitive abilities."*

My high school record was not much better. It can best be summarized by my consistent Ds in Chemistry and Auto Mechanics. The
D in Auto Mechanics may have emanated from my kicking the tire
instead of using the pressure gauge when the teacher asked me to
record the air pressure! If I were to summarize my mediocre high
school record, I would say that I was fortunate that there was no category for the selection of the graduate least likely to succeed – which I
would have won, hands down.

At the University of Wisconsin

In the fall of 1946, I entered the University of Wisconsin at the Madison campus, in the College of Agriculture, intending to teach Agriculture to high school students. My mother suggested I attend UW Platteville where I would have a lower chance of flunking out. I persuaded her to let me try Madison. Had I entered Platteville, as luck would have it, I would not have become a physician.

Given my lackluster performance in junior and high school, I was surprised to be told by my university Chemistry teaching assistant that the student sitting next to me had been copying my answers during the traditional 6-weeks' Chemistry examination. It was a new experience for me to do well enough that anyone would want to copy my answers in any subject, especially Chemistry. This success in Chemistry convinced me to change my major from Agriculture Education to Chemistry at the beginning of my second year at the University.

By virtue of some quirk, I found myself in a chemistry class where all of my classmates were enrolled in the Pre-Med program. My thought was, if the health of the citizens of Wisconsin was dependent on these classmates, I better help them, and I therefore changed my major again between semesters of my second year, this time from Chemistry to Pre-Med. Naturally, this required taking classes in one summer school session to offset my credits in Agronomy and Animal Husbandry, which were not transferable as Pre-Med requirements.

These early Pre-Med years were sprinkled with other occasional triumphs of cunning, if not intellect. In French class, which I attended along with my sister Janice, a Language major two years older than I, I happened to receive an A+++ on a writing assignment. Janice's grade was an A, without the plusses. To this day, she attributes my higher grade to my paper's description of our instructor as tres beau (very beautiful).

I was fortunate to live at the home of my parents in Cottage Grove during the seven years of Pre-Medical and Medical School. There were other expenses: tuition, books, clothing as well as limited entertainment expenses which I paid for from full-time summer jobs and part-time work during the school months. My main summer job was with the Kautz Construction Company erecting cement foundations for houses and other buildings.

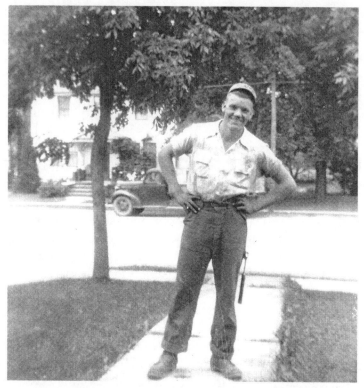

Summer job with Kautz Construction Co. (1948)

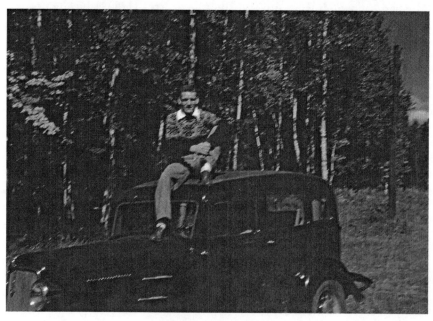

My first car (1951)

One summer a friend and I drove to Southern Nebraska to obtain employment by shocking bundles of grain in the fields. Fringe benefits included our meals and the privilege of sleeping in the farmer's barn. Salary was calculated on the basis of one dollar per acre shocked.

As the season progressed we traveled northward into South Dakota. I particularly remember attending a dance in Huron, South Dakota on a Saturday night and "dancing up a storm" in my circular striped T-shirt. Further north travels took us though North Dakota to the Canadian border during which time there were no more dances.

My part-time jobs during school were diverse: setting bowling pins, working in the University Student Union Rathskellar and driving a Checker cab during my 3rd year of Pre-Med and the first three years of Medical School.

One first for this previously mediocre student came from Dean Mark Ingraham:

THE UNIVERSITY OF WISCONSIN
COLLEGE OF LETTERS AND SCIENCE

February 7, 1950

Mr. Herbert F. Sandmire
Cottage Grove, Wisconsin
Dear Mr. Sandmire.

I am very happy to learn that you have been awarded Sophomore Honors in the College of Letters and Science at the completion of the first half of your four-year course.

This year you are in the top 6.5 per cent of the sophomore class. The list of the names of students winning these honors, appropriately framed, is hung on the south wall of the central corridor on the first floor of Bascom Hall.

Our rapidly changing world requires educated men and women. There is a growing need for scholarship in every field of endeavor. The existence of our civilization depends on keen intellect used strenuously for the good of humanity. Your record for the past two years has been distinguished. The University confidently expects that in the years to come you will exemplify its greatest contribution to mankind, the citizen of trained intelligence.

Sincerely yours,

Mark H. Ingraham, Dean of the College of Letters and Science

Perhaps I would not be the high school graduate least likely to succeed!

I did not tell my parents about the change of my major as there was no guarantee that I would be accepted by any medical school. Nevertheless, I received A's in all the rest of my courses after my major was changed to Pre-Med, and I was accepted into the University of Wisconsin Medical School in the fall of 1949. The letter came from the Dean of the Medical School, himself.

At the University of Wisconsin Medical School

THE UNIVERSITY OF WISCONSIN MEDICAL SCHOOL

June 27, 1949
Mr. Herbert F. Sandmire
Cottage Grove, Wisconsin
Dear Mr. Sandmire
I am pleased to inform you that the Admissions Committee has acted favorably upon your application for admission to the University of Wisconsin Medical School in September 1949. This acceptance is conditioned upon the completion of the following courses during the summer with grades of B or above:
Physics 1b
English Literature
Due notice will be given you as to registration and materials.
May I ask you to indicate your acceptance of this place in the Medical School before July 10, and to keep this office notified of any change of address.
Sincerely,
Wm. S. Middleton, M.D., Dean

William S. Middleton, the formidable dean of the Medical School, had both a national and international reputation. He had been the dean since 1935, except for a few years when he served as a General in the Army Medical Corps during World War II. He not only knew every one of the 70 medical students in each of the last two years by name, but also by their nicknames, which he had usually tagged them with on the basis of a wrong answer they had given to one of his questions. He continued his full teaching schedule despite the administrative requirements of his deanship. He was a strict disciplinarian, but in a manner that allowed (many would say required) respect from his students. His main goal for his students was to have their future patients receive the best possible care. That being the case, he was naturally opposed to medical students working at outside jobs during the school months.

As such, my job with the Checker Cab Company presented a bit of a risk to my standing in medical school. As luck would have it, while driving the cab one night at approximately 10 PM, I was instructed by the dispatcher to pick up Dr. and Mrs. Middleton at the Chicago and Northwestern train station. Having an awareness of his attitude on medical students working, I greeted this assignment with alarm. There was no escape available to me. As I approached the station, I spied the Middletons, (I can still see them to this day) together with their luggage, in front of the station. I immediately pulled my taxi cap even lower over my eyes as I pulled up to the curb. I got out of the cab, opened the trunk, placed their luggage in and was relieved that I had not been recognized – so I thought. With my cap still in the low position, I drove the Middletons to their West-side home, just off from Monroe Street. Just as I was closing the trunk, after removing their luggage, and still with my cap in the down position I heard the dreaded words that I feared most: "SANDMIRE, YOU KNOW WHAT I THINK ABOUT MEDICAL STUDENTS WORKING." My response, as always with a comment from Dr. Middleton, was: "Yes, sir." What I should have said, but didn't, was something I use to this day: "We have to eat."

Because of my work and school schedules, dating was somewhat infrequent. One of my occasional dates was Emily, who resided at Elizabeth Waters Hall. As it happened, I had a few dates with her, one of which was memorable, not because of her social skills or physical beauty but by my getting into trouble with the university police. Toward the end of that date, and while driving my mother's Studebaker, we decided to visit the Arboretum – a nature preserve on the southwest side of Madison. Normally, visitors to the Arboretum for a study of nature, do so during the daylight hours. While parked on a slight reverse incline, and "during our discussion of current world affairs," a vigorous rainstorm visited the area. About an hour later, we discovered that we were literally "stuck in the mud," not being able to get sufficient traction to climb up the slight incline. We stayed all night in my mother's car, waiting for the morning to arrive. As it turned out, Emily was reported as missing by her dormitory roommate. This prompted an investigation, led by a university police officer, Joe Hammersly, which initially involved interviews with some of my medical school classmates to determine if any of my past behaviors would indicate the possibility of my kidnapping Emily. Fortunately, with the sun out and a gentle breeze, the mud under Mom's car dried out, and with improved traction we were able to escape our entrapment. I dropped Emily off at her dormitory and headed to class, where my classmates told me that I was wanted by the university police.

Officer Joe Hammersly vigorously cross-examined me. "Why didn't I call?" he asked. "I needed to stay in the car to protect Emily," I answered.

After a few other questions, and with his vast relief that Emily had not been kidnapped, he merely sighed, "If it ever happens again, try your best to call us!!!!!" Where were cell phones when we needed them?

While in Medical School, two of my classmates belonged to the Three Squares Eating Club located in the basement of the First United Methodist Church, across the street from the Chemistry building. George Woodington and Louie Philipp would invite me occasionally for evening meals at a small cost to myself. Actually, I had more than eating in mind when I was invited. My ulterior motive was to check out the girls. I was particularly attracted to Crystal Ainsworth from Shawano, Wisconsin and Marbie Bryan from Kansas. As it would happen, Louie fixed me up for a blind date with who I thought was to be Marbie. Lo and behold, when I knocked on the door to pick up my blind date, Crystal appeared (I mixed up both the girl and the location!). I avoided looking surprised or hesitant in any way, asking if she was ready. She was and off we went.

During the next several months, I was dating alternately Crystal and Marbie. The particular girl in current favor could be identified as the one wearing my green ski sweater (a gift from my older sister Corinne). One of the two complained that the other stretched the sweater! As time went on, Crystal seemed to win the race for the "prize" – me. During the "courting," our usual date involved picking up Crystal in my Checker Cab and having a quick spaghetti dinner at Jimmy's Italian Restaurant just off South Park Street.

The Checker Cab Company ran meter cabs, as opposed to zone cabs. With a meter cab you were only allowed to take one party at a time to its destination, and they were charged the amount as determined by the meter, the handle of which must be turned to the down position. One evening as I picked up Crystal in my cab for a little social interaction, and as we were parked in the cab stand in front of the Park Hotel, I noticed a Checker cab pulling in next to us that was driven by Mr. Robert Bender, the Checker Cab Company's owner.

As you might assume, we were not permitted to have non-paying riders in our cab. Mr. Bender could see the meter flag was still in the up position, which would not be the case with a paying passenger. I saw him pick up his radio microphone and send (I assumed) a call to the dispatcher. Following this, I immediately received the dispatcher's call, "Checker 14. Do you have a passenger? 10-4."

I responded, "I do not have a passenger."

Bender again picked up his microphone and sent another message, after which I got another call from the dispatcher, "Checker 14, do you have a rider?"

My response was, "Yes, I do have a rider." Again, Bender picked up his microphone and sent another message, after which the dispatcher ordered me "to get rid of her." I may have followed the dispatcher's order that night, but today, 61 years later, I still have Sweetie by my side.

Wedding bells

Crystal Ainsworth and I were married September 15, 1951 between my second and third year of medical school and after her second year at the university. We lived upstairs in my folks' house, and both of us commuted to Madison (Crystal to work and I to Med School). She discontinued her education and became employed by the Student Employment Bureau. But not to be denied, 29 years later, in 1980, and after raising five children, she earned her degree from the University of Wisconsin-Green Bay.

Another interesting part of my last year of medical school was the four weeks we spent in Chicago, two weeks delivering babies for the Chicago Maternity Center and two weeks at the Chicago Lying-In Hospital. The standard practice at the Maternity Center was to work in pairs with another senior medical student who had already been there a week. The other student was in charge for the first week and then for the second week, I would be in charge of the delivery team with a new senior student joining me.

The Maternity Center offered a home delivery service that was conducted by senior medical students while prenatal care was provided at the Center office. Sleeping quarters for the medical students was a very large open area above a store with multiple cots and one bathroom for approximately ten students. There was one curtained off, private area which my wife and I occupied when she came to Chicago over the New Years weekend of 1953. She accompanied us at the home deliveries. I remember a baby was coming during the 1953 Rose Bowl game while Alan Ameche, Wisconsin's All-American running back, was running toward the goal line. The radio announcer described this, at the precise time I was calling in the report of our successful delivery. With my mind on Alan Ameche, I dutifully reported to the Maternity Center, the successful delivery of a newborn boy. Crystal interrupted me during the call, correcting me by indicating that the baby was really a girl! The maternity service offered an excellent, though unsupervised, learning experience and most importantly allowed us to pretend that we were already real doctors.

My medical school record was above average but not particularly outstanding. I graduated in May of 1953 and joined the United States Air Force with an assignment to report to the William Beaumont Army Hospital for my internship. We had junked our 1934 Plymouth and drove to El Paso in a nice 1949 Ford, recently purchased from one of Crystal's former boyfriends. During my internship I had the opportunity to analyze my own abilities compared with 20 other interns from 20 different medical schools. I felt, by that comparison, I had received a good medical school education. This was also supported by the positive feedback I received from faculty members at the completion of each of my internship rotations.

CHAPTER 2

Family members

MY MOTHER'S NUMBER one accomplishment in life was nurturing her nine children, making sure that they had enough to eat and affordable clothing. Above all, she provided a constant stimulus for us to do well in school. She recognized the importance for each of her nine children to have the best education that they were capable of achieving.

She inspired three of her daughters to emulate herself and become teachers: Cardell, born in 1917, became a grade school teacher; Corinne, born in 1919, and Janice, born in 1927, became high school teachers. After a few years, Cardell discontinued teaching and worked in a factory in Racine Wisconsin. After two years of teaching in Richland Center High School, Corinne joined the U.S. Army as a lieutenant, specializing in nutrition. Janice continued teaching Spanish at Sun Prairie until she reached retirement age. Unfortunately, Cardell, at age 92 had been suffering from advanced Alzheimer's disease for the past two years and passed away on October 6, 2010. Corinne, at age 91, is in good health, lives alone in her own home and drives her car to purchase groceries. (This was written eight months before she passed away at age 92 on the February 17, 2011). Janet, born in 1931 and the youngest of my four sisters, attended the University of Wisconsin at the Madison campus and worked as a social worker until her retirement.

It overwhelms me just to think of my mother's daily schedule attending to the needs for a family of eleven: preparing three meals a day, doing the laundry almost daily, hanging the clothes on a outdoor line to dry (winter or summer), frequently mending worn-out clothes, managing a large garden to ensure a sufficient year-around food supply (I remember one year her mentioning that she had canned 500 quarts of tomatoes), assisting several kids with homework, and urging them to do well. One job she did not have was cleaning the bathroom – our low-maintenance outhouse was easy to keep in a tidy condition. Considering her schedule, she must have, by the end of each day, been exhausted. And yet I never once asked her, "Mom, are you tired?" Like most children, I took her hard work for granted.

In the days before Wal-Mart superstores, providing food was a very different endeavor. Potatoes and carrots were kept in the cellar, string beans, peas and tomatoes were canned in two-quart jars, cabbage was converted to sauerkraut and kept in a large barrel in the cellar, and beef, pork and chicken were available whenever needed by butchering the animals and storing the cut-up parts in a commercially available freezer. This also applied to the deer meat which we got from my father's deer-hunting trips to the North woods.

In 1941, after her ninth child was in first grade, and with only five kids still living at home, Mother resumed her teaching career, taking a position in a one-room, grade one through eight school a few miles northeast of Sun Prairie, Wisconsin. As I mentioned earlier, my parents knew nothing about my switch from chemistry to a pre-med major until I showed them my acceptance letter from Dr. Middleton. By that time, I was less humble (earlier in my school years, I had much to be humble about) and was exceedingly proud of my accomplishments. I was finally able to reward my mother for the patience she had shown for this twenty-year old son who was about to enter medical school and become a physician – the pride I had stemmed from the pride she felt on that day she attended my graduation from medical school.

Just seven months later, my mother, at age fifty-five, died while we were in El Paso. She had rheumatic heart disease with atrial fibrillation resulting in a fatal stroke. I caught a ride on an Air Force flight to attend her funeral. Since Crystal was eight months pregnant with Cheryl, she could not come with me. Struck with sorrow, I found solace in the fact that my mother's short life was long enough to see her wayward son make good.

My father was born in Sylvan Township, Richland County, Wisconsin on November 25, 1897. He passed away in Fort Myers, Florida on April 6, 1983 at the age of 85. Prior to 1945, he was a tenant farmer renting approximately seven or eight different farms during that time period.

As stated previously, he had moved his family to Cottage Grove, Wisconsin in 1941 to be closer to the University of Wisconsin, eight miles away in Madison. He successfully operated the Clark farm until

1945 and then became the farm reporter, first for the *Stoughton Currier Hub* and then for Madison's *Capital Times*. After a few years he became a sales manager for the Blaney Seed Corn Company located in Madison. My father, with very little education, seemed to be good at whatever he did, be it farming, newspaper reporting or selling seed. His main passions were deer hunting and traveling.

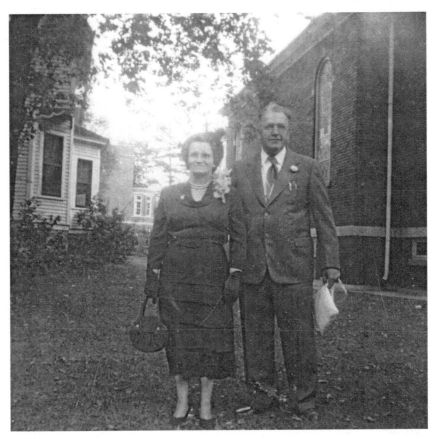

My parents, Glen and Bernadine Sandmire (1951)

My oldest brother Jim survived the Battle of the Bulge in Europe in December of 1944 at a time when the German army launched their last major offensive of World War II. Jim owned and operated a tavern right up to the time of his death from a heart attack on December 21, 1988 at age 68. He was well known for his good sense of humor. One of his favorites was to bluntly ask anyone who came to a function in an older automobile, "Was anyone hurt in that wreck?"

My next oldest brother Art's education ended at eighth grade. He worked in the Madison Oscar Mayer meat-packing plant for more than 40 years prior to his retirement 20 years ago. He has been a resident in a nursing home following a stroke two years ago, but with the help of walker he can still walk.

Cameron, nicknamed Ty, has operated a farm that includes a family campground. He has always had several riding horses as well as a team of Clydesdales as an added attraction at his campground. My youngest brother LaVaughn moved out of Wisconsin more than forty years ago and has maintained almost no contact with other family members.

I have been blessed with a wonderful upbringing, parents, and siblings, but there is no one more special to me than my bride, Crystal, who has been with me through all of the best and the worst of times, unwavering in her love, support, and companionship.

In 1981 Robert DeMott was serving his preceptorship under my direction in Green Bay and living at our house. During one weekend he brought his fiancée Susan to Green Bay to discuss with Crystal the life of being the wife of an obstetrician. Her abrupt answer was discouragingly short: "If you want to live your life as a single parent." Despite the advice Sweetie gave, Bob did become an obstetrician and Susan did marry him, probably on the basis of a hormonal connection. In 1987 Bob joined our practice at Ob-gyn Associates of Green Bay, Ltd.

"Sweetie" is the bond that has kept our family together throughout the years. Because of my heavy work schedule, she really was a "single parent" for much of the time, and, remarkably, while raising five kids, she resumed her quest for a university degree by enrolling in classes at University of Wisconsin-Green Bay. In December of 1980, she finally marched across the stage to Chancellor Weidner, received a kiss on the cheek and her diploma. I told her that she alone received the Weidner peck as she was old enough to spare Weidner a child molestation charge!

In July of 1986 she received the "Outstanding Member Award" from the Brown County Medical Society Auxiliary. Ann Lulloff, then Auxiliary President, wrote to me asking for any additional activities or talents she possessed. My response is scanned in:

April 13, 1986

Dear Herb,

This is the list of Crys' activities as we have them on file. Please add or delete as needed to make the list correct.

Brown County Medical Auxiliary

1967-68	Assistant Social Chairman	1974-75	Auditor
1968-69	Social Chairman	1975-76	"
1969-70	AMA-ERF Chairman	1976-77	"
1970-71	Sunshine Chairman	1977-78	"
1971-72	Archives-Historian	1981-82	"
1972-73	Treasurer	1983-84	President Elect
1973-74	Treasurer	1984-85	President

First United Methodist Church

Circle Member- Chairman of Nominating Committee- Member Board of Trustees

PEO

Has held all offices in organization including the presidency for 2 years

Zero Population

YWCA

Bellin Jr. Auxiliary- sustaining Member

Service League and Service League Auxiliary

UWGB Founders Association

Executive Committee, 2 years-Secretary 1983-84- Capital Fund Drive 1985

Scholarships Inc.-Board member many years-Chairman selections committee 2 years-
President 2 years

Fund drive Heritage Hill 1984-Member of Heritage Hill Guild

University League

Neville Public Museum Capital Fund Drive 1981-Chairman of one of 5 major
divisions

Family Service Association-Board of Directors 1983-85

Corporate Board Bellin Hospital-1984-85

Bellin Hospital Board of Trustees-1984-85

Served as a foster parent for a severley handicapped 16 year old and provided housing for him for one school year.

Letter from Ann Lulloff (1986)

Provided housing(in our home) for fourth year medical students from UW Madison
who were in Green Bay on their preceptorships from 1966-1985.
This certainly is an impressive list of accomplishments and you can be
very proud of Crys which I know you are. I would like to have the corrected
list back by the 25th of April. Thank you very much for your help, Herb.
Please keep this a secret.

Yours truly,

Ann Lulloff
2520 Betty Ct.
Green Bay, Wi. 54301

Dear Ann,

Please note correction regarding Bellin College of nursing; other assorted past and/or current activities include:

Carpenter
child Psychologist
landscape artist
Bicycle repair person
Plumber
Computer technologist
copywriter
Electrician
library resource person
Editorial consultant
legal assistant
motorcycle mechanic
Travel agent
adult Psychologist (street Husb.)

Cement worker
guidance counsellor
Research assistant
Cleaning lady
Painter < Pictures / Houses
answering service
Administrative assistant
Naturalist
Proof reader
Bird watcher
Tree surgeon
lover

I am probably forgetting many others. Thanks for thinking of her. Sincerely, Herb F. Sandmire

My response to the Lulloff letter.

Dian Page, *Green Bay Press Gazette* reporter in her "Who's Who" article of July 28, 1986, succinctly captured Crystal's outstanding accomplishments at that time:

> **Dian Page. People,** *July 28, 1986,* Green Bay Press Gazette
> *Outstanding service to the community as well as to the Brown County Medical Society Auxiliary earned the "Outstanding Member" Award this year for Crystal Sandmire. It's the auxiliary's very special honor and is not awarded every year.*
>
> *Sandmire's community involvement reads like a "Who's Who."*
>
> *Why does she do everything she does? "I like to try new and different things... to keep my mind active. The community has been good to us and I think it's important to do something in return," she says.*
>
> *So she's gotten involved in capital fund drives for the University of Wisconsin-Green Bay Founders Association as a member of its executive committee, the Neville Public Museum and Heritage Hill State Park.*
>
> *She is vice president of the Bellin College of Nursing Board of Trustees and on the nominating committee of the Family Service Association Board of Directors.*
>
> *She's held every office in her P.E.O. Chapter, including the presidency for two years, and has served as president and board member of Scholarships Inc.*
>
> *During her years in the medical auxiliary, she's held many offices, including that of president in 1984-85, chairman of the scholarship committee for 1985-86, and director for 1986-87.*
>
> *She's been a member of Zero Population Growth, the Green Bay-DePere YWCA, the Service League of Green Bay and Service League Auxiliary and Bellin Junior Auxiliary.*
>
> *From 1978 to 1985, the Sandmire home has been open to fourth-year medical students from the UW-Madison who have their preceptorships in Green Bay, and she served as foster parent for a handicapped 16-year old boy.*
>
> *Sandmire is the wife of Herbert Sandmire MD and the mother of their five children.*

The Dian Page article was a comprehensive summary of her accomplishments up to 1986. Another honor came to her in 2006 as she and I shared the Chancellor's Award at the University of Wisconsin-Green Bay.

Beginning about that time (1986) I began to depend on her as an adminstrative assistent for the preparation of my presentations, manuscripts, preparing power point screens and data input relative to my expert witness work. She continues in that role at this time entering my handwritten pages of this book into the computer.

Furthermore, she has willingly traveled with me to all of the 62 trials, mostly out-of-state and including Melbourne, Australia, where I have provided expert witness testimony. She routinely sits in the back row of the Court room, and I jokingly tell her that her facial expressions are unlawfully sending messages to me regarding the quality of my testimony.

All of you who know Sweetie will understand how lucky I am to have gone to the "Three Squares Eating Club" more than 60 years ago for reasons other than obtaining a low-cost meal. I drew the long straw when I got hooked up with Sweetie. In addition to being multi-talented, as described in my letter to Ann Lulloff, her most important responsibility, in her opinion, was being a good mother. She was and still is a patient listener and counselor whenever any of our children seek her advice.

Cheryl, at 57 years of age, is the oldest of our children. She is an artist and photographer, having graduated with honors from Brooks Institute of Photography in Santa Barbara, California. Following her graduation, she was hired by "Brooks" as a teaching assistant. She has been very successful in her career and has received numerous photography awards. For the past several years she has owned and operated her own studio in Boise, Idaho. More recently she has traveled to Italy to do photography and develop the artistic aspect of her career.

Cheryl, at age 13, had been to a girlfriend's house three evenings in succession and therefore was told by her mother that she needed to stay home that evening. These circumstances resulted in Cheryl's decision to "run away." Her mother, at about 10pm, discovered Cheryl was not sleeping in her bed. I was, at that time, attending a labor patient at the hospital and received a call from Sweetie, in a near panic condition, reporting the missing "run-away delinquent." She wanted my advice as to her next step: call the police?; call people living in the neighborhood?; or call all of Cheryl's friends who lived in the neighborhood?.

I inquired about whether the other four little urchins could hear her (Sweetie's) side of the conversation? She said "yes," so I told her to announce in a loud voice: "Dad said to change all of the locks on the doors in case she took a key!" None of our other four kids ever decided to run away.

About one half hour after she was discovered missing, she returned from the home of her friend Missy Cherney, who lived just two blocks away.

Yvonne, in 1974, was one of the first college students to benefit from Title IX, a federal program that provided women with the same opportunities as men to participate in college sports and to receive athletic scholarships. Arizona State University offered, and she accepted, a full, four-year scholarship, and she became an all-conference gymnast. A short newspaper article describes her academic achievements: "Yvonne Sandmire, daughter of Dr. and Mrs. Herbert Sandmire, recently graduated from Arizona State University, Tempe, Arizona, with first honors. In addition she was nominated by the Athletic Department for 'Outstanding Student of the Year.' She also received 'Outstanding Student in the College of Communications" during the honors convocation."

She went on to coach the women's gymnastics team at Boise State University for 20 years. We saw Vonnie's team crowned as champions of the Western Gymnastics conference. The championship meet was hosted by her Boise State University team in Boise, Idaho. As parents we were exceedingly proud of her as we witnessed her receiving the trophy. We realize that being a successful coach in addition to having coaching skills involved being a role model, and having "parenting" and counseling skills. Actually her team had won prior conference championships five times since 1997.

Carla Chambers, team captain for the Broncos said,"Sandmire drives her team with her unbelievable optimism and unyielding enthusiasm. She is wild and happy which makes the team comfortable in competition." Yvonne is married to Cary Hattabaugh of Boise, Idaho. She and Cary have a son Trevor age 16.

Kevin, our oldest son, at age 54, is an internal medicine specialist in Green Bay and is married to Karen Budic. He attended the University of Wisconsin at Madison for both his undergraduate and medical degrees. As an undergraduate he was awarded membership in the honor societies of Phi Kappa Phi and Phi Beta Kappa. In addition, he was the recipient of the Vilas/Chancellor's Scholarship as well as the Mary Shine Peterson undergraduate scholarship for his outstanding work in biochemistry. He was named a Chancellor's Scholar for the 1975-76 school year. Kevin and Karen have two sons, Kyle and Kurt ages 20 and 23.

Michael, age 50, practices law in Portland, Oregon and is married to Lisa Brown. He was an honor student at Preble High School after which he attended Stanford University for both his undergraduate and law degrees. While at Stanford Law School he was an editor for the Stanford Law Journal. He currently is in line to become President of the Oregon Association of Defense Councils. Michael and Lisa have a son Andrew age 12 and identical twin sons Malcolm and Cameron ages 10.

David, age 47, has a medical degree and is a professor at the University of New England in Maine and is married to Beth Weir. He was also an honor student at Preble High School and attended the University of Wisconsin for his undergraduate degree where he was admitted to Phi Eta Sigma Freshman Honor Society and was placed on the Dean's list. He was also elected to Phi Beta Kappa, Phi Kappa Phi, and Golden Key National Honor Societies. He received his medical degree from the University of Wisconsin, Madison. He has been the recipient of numerous teaching awards during his career and has authored several scientific articles and one book. David and Beth have a son Alec age 19 and one daughter Crystie age 16 (our only granddaughter.

They are a great group of kids and have enriched our lives immensely. They got us to do things we would not have done on our own, and I might add will never do again, like white water rafting on the Snake River in Idaho and jumping in the hot springs of the Yellowstone River in mid-winter. In the latter case, we parked the car, walked about one half mile down a trail where we stripped down to our bathing suits with only a blanket protecting us from the snow below. This was tolerable as we soon slipped down an icy slope into the hot springs area in the river. This was very pleasant until we had to climb up the icy slope and get dressed in the frigid temperature, then trek one half mile back to our car. Exhilarating ???!!!

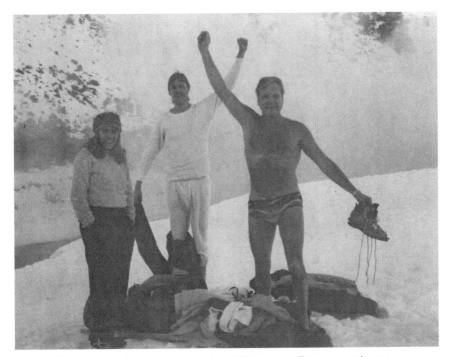

Swimming in hot springs in the Yellowstone River in mid-winter
(December 1985)

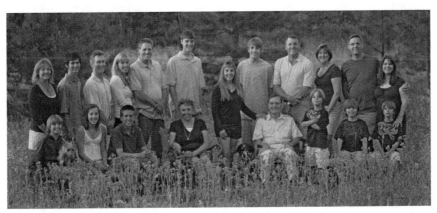

Sandmire family picture at Cheryl's Idaho cabin (July 2008)

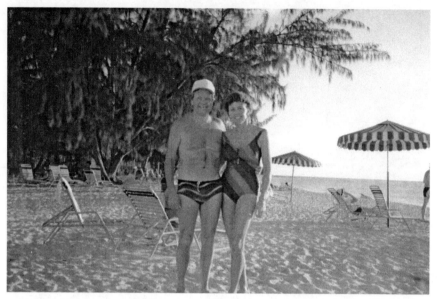

Working winter vacation on Grand Cayman Island (January 1984)

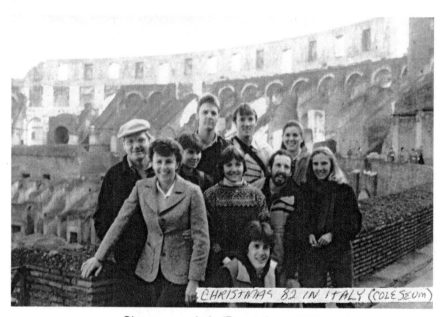

Christmas in Italy (December 1982)

CHAPTER 3

At the 5001st USAF hospital at Fairbanks, Alaska

FOLLOWING MY INTERNSHIP, I was assigned to the 5001st USAF base hospital at Fairbanks, Alaska. We drove back to Wisconsin (via North Carolina to visit my sister Corinne and her family) for leave time of four weeks prior to my travel to the West coast to ship our car and myself to Fairbanks. Crystal and baby Cheryl came six weeks later after I found housing.

The Korean War ended in 1953, but the doctor draft continued a few more years. My purpose in selecting a military internship was to get into the service without the delay of waiting to be drafted. With the Korean War over, the three trained obstetricians at our 5001st USAF Base Hospital were due to be discharged within six months and replaced by non-obstetrically trained general medical officers. As a general medical officer, I was given a crash course in the performance of forceps and cesarean deliveries. Within six months of my assignment to that hospital I was, at 25 years of age, the chief of an obstetric service delivering 125 babies a month.

The two years experience at the Air Force Hospital was particularly rewarding and helped me hone all of the skills needed to be a good obstetrician. In fact, for any two-year period during my entire professional career, I would rate the Fairbanks experience as the best. Part of the joy of life in Fairbanks was our interaction with fellow physicians and their families, now in a more relaxed manner compared to medical school and internship. Dr. Daitch, one of our "obstetricians," became a father during his stay at Ladd Air Force Base Hospital. I was privileged to become the godfather of his newborn son during the circumcision ceremony-all decked out in my yarmulke, Jewish skull cap.

On October 23, 1955 we had a patient who was vigorously bleeding following her delivery. She had afibrinogenemia resulting from amniotic fluid infusion. We had the foresight to have fibrinogen available for a condition that had only been reported in the literature two years earlier by Reid, Weiner and Roby. Our diagnosis and successful treatment of this patient resulted in it being submitted and accepted for publication as a case report in the September 1956 issue of the *United States Armed Forces Medical Journal*.

In severe cases of afibrinogenemia, with the large amounts of the amniotic fluid that normally surround the fetus entering the mother's circulation, a violent reaction occurs similar to severe allergic anaphylactic shock. The lungs of the mother rapidly become non-functional, and blood fails to clot, resulting in the rapid bleeding from a large number of sites. The failure of the blood to clot is due to the inadequate levels of fibrinogen, one of the essential components needed for normal clotting. The available circulating fibrinogen is rapidly used up by formation of intravascular clots that line all of the mother's blood vessels.

One portal of entry of amniotic fluid into the mother's circulation may be through the exposed veins in the cervix that can be torn during labor. Rupture of the membranes early in labor may expose these veins to considerable amounts of amniotic fluid. The condition worsens if the baby's head blocks the cervix, causing an increase in pressure within the uterus. Without the normal amount of circulating fibrinogen, clot formation at the former attachment of the afterbirth, and all other raw areas, does not take place, resulting in vigorous bleeding following the delivery. Our patient lost about two of her five quarts of blood. Her pulse rose to 120 and blood pressure fell to shock levels of 70/50 mm Hg. Her blood obtained for cross matching for transfusion had failed to clot in the test tube, thereby confirming our working diagnosis of afibrinogenemia. At that point we gave her two grams of fibrinogen, which dramatically decreased her vaginal bleeding.

As our case report noted, "Our patient was treated in an isolated station hospital about 2000 miles from a commercial source of fibrinogen. We were fortunate in having fibrinogen on hand and we hope that this case report will stimulate other military hospitals to procure this important drug."

While I could not have imagined it at the time, this represented the first of what would eventually be 47 scientific papers, 27 letters to the editor and six miscellaneous articles that I have published. *What possessed this 26-year old general medical officer (not specialty trained) to believe he could make a contribution to the medical literature?*

Who determines which articles get published in a peer-reviewed journal?

Perhaps this is a good place to describe the "road to publication" process. The editor, together with the journal's editorial board, will make the final decision to accept or reject all articles submitted by authors for publication. The editor typically assigns three reviewers to review each article for potential reader interest, the correctness of the methodology, the accuracy of the findings, and the statistical significance or lack thereof for each of the reported results. The reviewers are chosen by the editor on the basis of having demonstrated expert knowledge of the issues involved in the submitted paper and having published research findings on the same or a similar subject. The reviewers' evaluations and recommendations are the most important determinant in judging the article's suitability for publication. During the course of my professional career I have served as an editorial reviewer for several publications, including *Obstetrics and Gynecology*, the *American Journal of Obstetrics and Gynecology*, *Birth*, the *New England Journal of Medicine*, the *International Journal of Gynecology and Obstetrics*, the *Wisconsin Medical Journal*, and the *Journal of Hand and Microsurgery* (in India).

One satisfying part of the Fairbanks experience involved my moonlighting, part-time job for a local general surgeon, Henry Storres. Actually, I was performing a cesarean delivery for Dr. Storres at St. Joseph's Hospital in downtown Fairbanks during the time that our second child, Yvonne, was born. The temperature that morning, January 11, 1956, was minus 53 degrees Fahrenheit. The Air Force hospital was just one and one half blocks from our base-housing, but with that temperature tires freeze, leaving insufficient traction to get out of the depressed area which results from the snow falling on top of the car and not below it. With headbolt heaters the car started, but we could not move it. I took our daughter Cheryl to a neighbor and then walked Crystal to the hospital. From there I called a taxi for my trip downtown. After I completed the cesarean delivery, I called the Ladd Air Force Hospital to find that Yvonne had already arrived. *Talk about an efficient laborer!*

During the 1950s, the population of Fairbanks was approximately 10,000. There were no real recreational facilities in the area except for bowling alleys and ski hills – used by us only if it was warmer than 20 below zero. Actually I was on two bowling teams and substituted on a third, the dental team. With all of the darkness and cold, bowling provided a welcomed distraction. As the only officer on the hospital bowling team, I had the lowest average, meaning I was the poorest bowler. Despite my mediocrity, our hospital team won the Ladd Air Force Base Championship one year. I have a trophy to prove it.

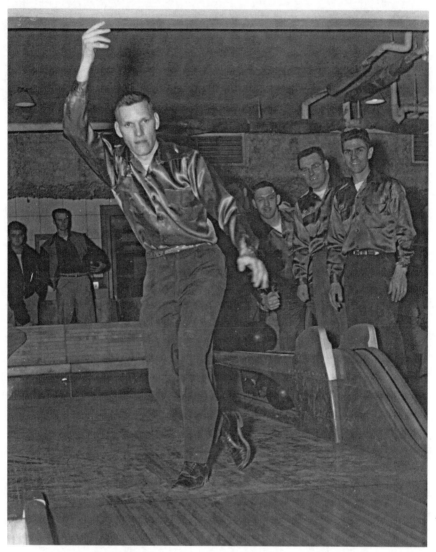

The "Champion Bowler" who wasn't !! (1955)

Skiing was tolerable if the temperature was higher than 20 below zero but involved going to the lodge following every other trip down the hill to warm up before venturing out for the next run. The isolation of living in the Alaskan wilderness certainly prodded us to try things we hadn't done before. Still, my short bowling career was never resumed after leaving Fairbanks and the Air Force on the 30th of June 1956. The same can be said for my brief stint hunting caribou. We went hunting on the 18th of October 1954 in 18 below zero weather. This also was a "one-shot" successful activity for me. We had no need to take our caribou carcass to be frozen or to keep it frozen - we simply placed it in one of our spare upstairs bedrooms with the window open. By June when the warm weather appeared, we had consumed all of the caribou meat.

Survival in the frozen tundra was part of our Air Force Alaska training and experience. We rode out to a remote area on trucks, set up our tents, got into sleeping bags and slept! If it became colder than 30 degrees below zero we were brought back to our warm quarters. We all prayed for the temperature to go down to that threshold level. Our prayers were answered and we had a shortened survival experience.

In Fairbanks, the length of daylight sunshine ranged from one hour on January 31st to more than 23 hours on June 20th. The Air Base routinely scheduled a softball game to start at midnight without artificial lights on June 20th of each year.

"Cabin fever" was an "illness" indigenous to the Fairbanks area and seemed to afflict those of us from the "States" (Alaska was not yet a state) after tolerating two Fairbanks' winters. Symptoms included frustration, irritability and a lack of cheerfulness (even for one known for cheerfulness).

CHAPTER 4

Choosing a residency

FOLLOWING MY EYE-OPENING experience as an "obstetrician" at Ladd Air Force Base Hospital, I knew more about obstetrics than family practice or any other specialty. Therefore, it was natural for me to consider a career in obstetrics and gynecology. I knew nothing about which residency programs were top-notch and which were not. Consequently, I applied first at the University of Wisconsin. John Harris, founding chairman of the Department of Obstetrics and Gynecology had passed away about two years before and had been replaced by interim Chairperson, Dr. Ralph Campbell, 3rd President of the American Academy of Obstetrics and Gynecology, forerunner of the American College of Obstetrics and Gynecology (ACOG). Astonishingly, he wrote back informing me that they were filled with applicants for the next two years. I told Crystal that he must have obtained my high school records.

Nevertheless, I asked Crystal about what medical schools we could consider which were close to Wisconsin. She mentioned the University of Iowa, and I decided to apply there. What I did not know at that time, but what I became aware of over subsequent years, was that the Iowa obstetrics and gynecology residency was outstanding in comparison to many other programs. I got lucky, yet again. In fact, I was accepted by the chairman of the Iowa program, Dr. John Randall, even before he had received the letter of recommendation from General Maxwell, outlining, in a glowing fashion, my accomplishments at Ladd Air Force Base Hospital:

State University of Iowa
Department of Obstetrics and Gynecology
December 15, 1955

Dr. Herbert F. Sandmire
5001ˢᵗ USAF Hospital,
APO 731, Seattle, Washington.
Dear Doctor Sandmire:
Your letter of the 9ᵗʰ of December has been received. We will be very happy to have you as one of our residents starting July 1, 1956. In the near future you will receive a letter from Superintendent Hartman giving you general information about your residency, such as information about your salary, board and room, and laundry.

If there is anything I can do for you between now and July 1ˢᵗ, please feel free to write to me.

I hope that you have a very Merry Christmas and a pleasant New Year.

Very truly yours,
J.H.Randall, M.D.,
Professor and Head,
Department of Obstetrics and Gynecology.

State University of Iowa
Department of Obstetrics and Gynecology
Iowa City, Iowa
December 19, 1955

Brigadier Gen. Earl Maxwell,
Headquarters Alaskan Air Command,
APO 942, Seattle, Washington.
Dear Doctor Maxwell:
Thank you very kindly for your letter on behalf of Doctor Sandmire. He has already been given a residency in our Department but nevertheless we are pleased to have your opinion of him.

Very truly yours,
J.H.Randall, M.D.,
Professor and Head,
Department of Obstetrics and Gynecology

Having delivered more than 100 babies during my internship and approximately 800 more in my two years at Ladd Air Force Hospital, I had much more experience than the other residents in the department.

Nonetheless, it was important for me, despite my vast pre-residency experience, to conduct myself in a humble fashion in my relationship with the other residents, especially those more senior to me in the residency hierarchy. Generally speaking, I believe I had a good relationship with all the other obstetrics and gynecology residents.

Housing in Iowa City

We had signed up for University housing, which involved moving into World War II quonset "apartments." Following the second week in that setting, with one quonset building being no more than a foot from others on each end, we determined that we had to move. Borrowing $400 from Crystal's Aunt Inez for the down payment, we bought a small house that was built on a cement slab with no basement. It did have three small bedrooms, one about the size of a large closet. Monthly payments were $75 compared to $45 to rent the quonset "apartment." Three years later we sold our small house at a $1000 profit and paid off the mortgage balance as well as Crystal's aunt.

On December 14, 1956, five weeks before his due date, our son Kevin was delivered by cesarean section performed by Iowa's Dr. John Randall, Chief of the Obstetrics and Gynecology Department. The complication requiring the cesarean birth was called placenta previa, meaning the placenta was located too low in the uterus, resulting in brisk uterine bleeding. Kevin developed severe respiratory distress a few hours after birth that lasted several days, resulting in a pessimistic outlook for his survival by both of his grandfathers, one of which later admitted thinking "that boy would never live."

CHAPTER 5

The urge to publish and practice
with Dr. Austin

IT WAS DURING my residency years that I was severely bitten by the "publication bug," resulting in my second paper, "Ectopic Pregnancy – A review of 182 cases," published in the August 1959 issue of *Obstetrics and Gynecology*. The presentation of this paper in September of 1958 at the annual meeting of ACOG's District VI in Des Moines, Iowa resulted in my being the recipient of my first award: First Place Residents' Paper Award. My own analysis, at that time, was that those who have been bitten by the publication bug and have published research studies, generally do so in order "to make a difference" for other physicians and more importantly for other physicians' patients. Not all of my colleagues share my take on this - one cynic has described an expert as an "asshole out of town with slides."

The major pearls (medical jargon for important findings and recommendations) of my second article were as follows: 1) Twenty nine of 182 received an incorrect diagnosis. 2) Nine of 29 would have had the correct diagnosis made, had a colpocentesis (a puncture through the vagina, behind the uterus to determine the presence of internal bleeding into the abdominal cavity) been performed. 3) One hundred eleven of 182 had a colpocentesis performed with a true positive finding in 99 (89%). 4) Colpocentesis was highly recommended as its use resulted in the correct diagnosis in 89% of the cases where it was performed.

During the summer of 1959, I used my three-week vacation time to fill in for a private obstetrician in Marion, Indiana, while he was recovering from surgery. We drove to Marion and Crystal, with our three very young children in tow, took the train to her parent's farm in

Shawano, Wisconsin. Our Iowa City neighbors, when hearing of our plans, offered Crystal some tranquilizers to prevent anxiety at the time of their changing trains in Chicago. Not knowing their possible effect, she did not take or need them. The train trip was a new and intimidating experience for the children, who were afraid to walk in the swaying train from their coach to the dining car. They lost their appetites and refused to eat once they got to the dining car. When Crystal's parents picked them up at the train station in Shawano, they marveled at the fact that each of the little kids was carrying their own little suitcase. The Marion experience for me was professionally and financially rewarding and again allowed me to pretend to be a real obstetrician.

With my residency completed, I considered and was interviewed at three separate practices: the Sheboygan Clinic, the Appleton Medical Arts Clinic, and the office of Dr. Stephen (Drake) Austin in Green Bay. Desiring more independence in my practice, I decided to avoid the clinics and signed on with Dr. Austin starting July 13th, 1959. This was ironic because four years later, I started recruiting Green Bay doctors to join in the formation of the Beaumont Clinic, which opened in June of 1965.

My starting salary with Dr. Austin was $900 per month and at my request was increased by $100 after the first six months. Dr. Austin, the only trained obstetrician in Green Bay and a solo practitioner for the previous five years, was happy to have me as a partner. Later in our association, I quizzed him about how he happened to choose me for his partner – he replied, "Herb, that was easy, there were no other applicants!"

Drake had obtained four Green Bay Packer season tickets and gave two of them to us. He was a bonified Packer fan, as demonstrated by his criticism of questionable calls by the officials. Another trait he had was to lean into the person seated next to him in the direction he wanted the Packer ball carrier to go. At six feet four inches and a weight of 230 pounds, he was able to generate considerable "leaning force."

Unfortunately, following a short illness due to lung cancer, Dr. Austin passed away. Below are remarks that I made at the Stephen Drake Austin Memorial service on November 26, 1986:

> *We are drawn together to celebrate the life of a remarkable man.*
> <u>*Who was Drake Austin?*</u>
> *To his colleagues: The leader of the Green Bay obstetrical community, a man nearing retirement but as interested in and as current on new developments within his specialty as new physicians, with 30 to 40 years of practice ahead of them.*

To his friends: A polite, considerate, intelligent man with a remarkable sense of humor.

To his patients: A man devoted to their needs, sincere in his administration of care and possessed with the patience of Job.

To his staff: A great boss; they had profound respect for his talents and accomplishments. Staff persons learned quickly his method of exhibiting exasperation when his patience was tried, which was to bend his head slightly forward, peer over the top of his glasses downward (always because of his stature) at the target person, and then followed a detonating silence – the look carried the message.

To me: Drake and I were remarkably different in background, education, recreational pursuits, dress, and at times, political persuasion. In spite of this, in 27 ½ years of sharing our patients and thoughts, we never had an important difference. The closest thing to a significant difference was his recurring admonition: "Herb, only an idiot would ride a motorcycle!" Once proclaimed, I was left to consider whether there are disadvantages to being an idiot. Dr. Austin was loved by his patients and medical staff and respected by all who had the good fortune to know him.

To Rick: A good husband – must have been; Rick only informed me of a few peccadilloes. Rick, on Monday night, observed that she and I had something in common: He chose both of us. Choosing a partner can be a difficult task. Drake and I reflected on this very subject many years ago whereupon I asked him if he had experienced difficulty in choosing me as his partner. Being a man of few words, he responded, "No." This puzzled me. If he had special skills or advice on this process, I wanted him to share them with me. I inquired, "Why was it not difficult?" His reply was – "there were no other applicants." Were there other applicants when he chose Rick? This historian is not privy to that information.

There is a time and place for tears.

There is a time and place for acceptance.

This is the time and place to celebrate the life and special contributions of this remarkable man.

A note received from Rick during Drake's illness:

Dear Crys and Herb,

Thank you for the lovely basket and all of its goodies. Sometimes for lunch all Drake wants is a milk shake – so that elegant chocolate sauce is terrific!

Your kind words about our long association really moved us. Especially me. I wish the tears were not so close to the surface! We will never ever forget when you two arrived in Green Bay. Immediately the quality of life improved 150%. And it continues to be the greatest partnership and now the extended group. Really, so little of the irritations and fault-finding among "our guys."

Drake has re-entered Bellin for more diagnostic work-ups. Now he's to see a cardiologist. Thank you, Crys and Herb, for so many kindnesses over the years.   Love, Rick

CHAPTER 6

The Green Bay Packer Glory Years, 1959 - 1967

PRIOR TO COMING to Green Bay in 1959, I was aware of the Green Bay Packers but did not have sufficient interest to be considered a Packer fan. As you can see by my rather lengthy description of the Green Bay Packer Glory Years, 1959 – 1968, that rapidly changed during the Lombardi years. My wife and I have many fond memories of attending all of the home Packer games – only missing games if I had a patient in active labor. When doctors attending the Packer games were needed to provide care for a patient, they would be paged by their number over the public address system. The number I dreaded to hear was 490 - mine.

Packer Sunday was not only a great sports event; it was also a social event. Many fans entertained in their homes with pre-game and post-game parties. It was one long day of celebrating. Some of the parties were even reported in the *Green Bay Press Gazette* on the society page. Our local paper no longer has a society page.

Fans dressed more fashionably for the games back then. It was not uncommon to see many fur coats, fashionable boots and shoes. Today we consider comfort more than fashion. We participated in all this activity in a limited way as we did not want to leave our children with a sitter for such a long day.

The Packers and Bears were the only founding members (1919) of the National Football League (NFL) fielding teams in 1959. Over the years the Packers had become the powerhouse of the league, as evidenced by their five championships (1929, 1930, 1931, 1936 and 1944) in the first 25 years of the league play. By 1958, the Packers had reached a low point in their formerly illustrious 40-year history, with a season record of 1-10-1. Despite the eternal losing seasons during the 1950s, the Packers executive board and the Green Bay community were sufficiently optimistic to construct the new City Stadium in 1957 with a seating capacity of 32,150.

The Packers last (barely) winning season was 6-5-1, accomplished by the 1947 squad. During the 1950s three separate coaches, Gene Ronzani, Lisle "Liz" Blackbourn and finally 1958 coach Scooter McLean, tried, without coming close, to produceing a winning record. The 1958 team, as subsequent years would demonstrate, did not lack talented players. The squad included stalwarts Bob Skoronski, Ron Kramer, Dan Currie, Jerry Kramer as well as future Hall of Famers Bart Starr, Forrest Gregg, Jim Taylor and Paul Hornung.

Why did McLean fail? The consensus seems to be that his lack of leadership led to his failure to motivate his players. For example, he did not maintain a distance from his players or the media – often seen playing poker with members from each group. He lacked the will to discipline players and to set rules to be followed. I also believe he lacked the energy to be creative in mapping out game plans for his team. In short, he was not a true leader. In his defense, though, members of the Packers executive committee were known to put pressure on him on behalf of different players petitioning for more playing time, and he often found himself caught in the middle.

This could not happen under Vince Lombardi, who with the advice of Packer official, the late Jack Vanisi, held out for the general manager's role in addition to becoming coach. Furthermore, he wisely announced at the start of his tenure that he would not tolerate any interference from executive board members or anyone else in the way he coached the team or administered the franchise.

Lombardi became head coach and general manager of the Green Bay Packers at age 45, after having been passed over several times for other head coaching positions. In the three years prior to his becoming head coach, the Packers' record was 8-27-1 with a quarterback who wanted to but had not played regularly for the Lombardi predecessors. Bart Starr was extremely disappointed when Lombardi obtained quarterback Lamar McHan from the St. Louis Cardinals. Overall, Lombardi eliminated 15 of the 36 players from the 1958 squad in the process of constructing his 1959 team.

When asked by the media if he thought the players would be receptive to him, he interrupted the questioner and retorted, "I don't care what they think of me, they need to be concerned about what I think of them!" Similarly, at his first meeting with the players he declared, "Gentlemen, I have never been associated with a losing team, and I do not intend to start now."

Lombardi snookered Paul Brown, Cleveland coach, obtaining via the trade route Lew Carpenter, Bobby Freeman, Henry Jordan and Bill Quinlan. Additional trades brought "Fuzzy" Thurston (who had been cut by three other teams) from Baltimore and Emlen Tunnell and John Dittrich from the Giants. Rookie Boyd Dowler, a superb receiver out of Colorado, made the 1959 squad as well.

In the 1950s, the NFL players were overwhelmingly white with very few black players on the roster. Nate Borden, a Green Bay Packer member since 1955, remained the only black player on the roster through the 1957 season. The white players in the late 1950s and 1960s commonly brought their wives and children to Green Bay for the season or entire year. Bart and Cherry Starr, for example, moved to Green Bay permanently in the summer of 1957 because they saw Green Bay "as a quiet town with traditional values." Soon thereafter, they became members of the First United Methodist Church in Green Bay. Many other Packer players and their wives also joined the Methodist Church as we had when we arrived in Green Bay in July of 1959.

The wives of Packer players and coaches were commonly seen in our office for their gynecological care and deliveries, mainly because my senior partner, Dr. Austin, was the first and only obstetrician in Green Bay from 1954 until I joined him in 1959. As more African American players made the roster during the 1960s and thereafter, they tended to not bring their families to Green Bay, although there were some exceptions.

The 1959 Green Bay Packer season

Following their dismal 1958 season, tickets were readily available and thus we bought four children's tickets, subsequently converted to adult tickets, plus two adult tickets. We still have our original six tickets, but now the waiting period is calculated to be more than forty years for ticket applicants – and will likely be even longer in the aftermath of their recent victory in Super Bowl XLV. At the time of a ticket holder's death, the tickets are required to be returned to the Green Bay Packers unless they have been included in the deceased's will.

With Lombardi at the helm, the Packers became instant winners for the first time since 1947, victorious in four of their six exhibition games. The 1959 Packer season was memorable to me for many reasons, the most important of which was that I had become an avid fan by the time the 1959 regular season started. I was amazed at the degree of excitement I had in anticipation of each game.

Following the exhibition season, the Packers opened the regular season with a game against the hated rival Chicago Bears. The now two-year old City Stadium was packed with Packer fans (as was true, at the time of this writing, for every game during the next 51 years) excited about the anticipated change in fortune under the direction of new coach and general manager Vincent Lombardi. The home game against the Bears started the 1959 NFL season on September 27. The Packers, unbelievably, eked out a nine-to-six win, limiting the highly rated Bears (8-4 in 1958) to just two field goals. The Packers Jim Taylor scored the game's only touchdown, but the extra point try failed. The victory in this game made believers out of the ecstatic fans that the now 5-2 (including pre season games) record under the new coach was not a fluke and that it foreshadowed more victories to come.

The second game against the Detroit Lions, also at home, was won by the Packers, 28-10, with the help of LaMar McHan's four touchdown passes (with Bart Starr still waiting in the wings).

The Packers won their next game at San Francisco, 21-20. Increasingly confident Packer fans started to wonder if they were staring at an undefeated regular season. Their elation was quickly squelched, however, as the Packers lost the next five games, including a 45-6 drubbing by the Rams and a 38-21 loss to the Colts, dropping their record to 3 and 5. We avid fans in unison faced reality! But the pendulum swung again with the ninth game when the Packers defeated Washington 21-0 and then followed with a 24-17 win over the Lions during the traditional Thanksgiving Day game. In the eleventh game the Packers beat the Los Angeles Rams 38-20, and the following week they were victorious over the 49ers 36-14 for their first winning regular season record (7-5) in twelve years. We fans were again ecstatic, especially about the forthcoming 1960 season for which we had championship dreams.

The 1960 season

The Packers lost to the Bears in the opener 17-14 with Starr passing for only 77 yards. With McHan at quarterback, the Packers won the next three games. In game five Starr started the second half against the Pittsburgh Steelers, and the Packers pulled out a 19-13 victory. In game six Baltimore defeated the Packers 38-24. The following week the Packers trounced Dallas 41-7. The Packers lost to the Rams 33-31 and at Detroit 23-10 for a 5-4 record. With their revenge win over the

Bears by 41-13 there was a three-way tie with the Colts and 49ers for first place in the Western Conference at 6-4. In game eleven the Packers defeated the 49ers 13-0 while Baltimore lost to the Rams 10-3. Therefore, Green Bay was in first place with one game remaining, which they won 35-21 over the Rams to win their first conference championship since 1944. Back in Green Bay, the team plane was greeted by 15,000 fans.

The Philadelphia Eagles were the Eastern Conference champions with a 10-2 record while Green Bay was 8-4. The Eagles defense, thought to be marginal, was anything but in the NFL title game that was won by the Eagles 17-13. Lombardi's final statement to his 1960 squad was, "This will never happen again. You will never lose another championship." **He was right.**

The 1961 season

At the start of the 1961 season there were two changes in the NFL: 1) the Minnesota Vikings entered the league and 2) the regular season schedule was expanded to 14 games.

The 1961 Packers were undefeated in the exhibition games but again lost the opener, this time to the Lions 17-13 before 44,307 fans at Milwaukee County Stadium. During that time period the Packers played two or three regular season home games in Milwaukee County Stadium, a facility that was much larger than Green Bay City Stadium, which had a capacity of 32,500. This was also a way of showing appreciation to Milwaukee fans for their financial support during lean years of the Packers. Green Bay City Stadium eventually expanded to 70,000 and was renamed Lambeau Field in honor of Curly Lambeau, founder of the Packers. Today, the Milwaukee fans are given the option of purchasing two home game tickets, but all games are played in Green Bay.

Rebounding from the Detroit loss, the Packers won the next three games against strong opponents by a combined score of 49-17, largely because of a dominant defense. The fifth game was played before 75,000 Cleveland Brown fans in Municipal Stadium. Incidentally, Lombardi continued to snooker Cleveland coach Paul Brown by trading for Willie Davis, a future Hall of Famer and outstanding defensive end for the Packers over the next seven years. Not to be intimidated by the 75,000 rabid Brown's fans, the "Pack" destroyed Cleveland 49-17. Back to back wins over the new Minnesota Vikings provided a 6-1 record to close out the first half of the 1961 schedule. Things turned worse, though, when Jerry Kramer broke his ankle and Hornung,

Dowler and Nitschke were called up for duty by the National Guard during the Berlin crisis. As it turned out, only Nitschke and Kramer were unavailable to play.

The Pack got trounced by the Colts 45-21, bringing them to 6 and 2 for the season. They rebounded the next week against the Bears, winning 31-28. Bears Coach George "Papa Bear" Halas complained to his players in a sexist manner by claiming that they were "playing like girls." The Pack won the next three games, defeating the Rams, Lions and Giants, but split their last two games to finish as Western Division champions with an 11-3 record.

The Pack annihilated the New York Giants 37-0 in the NFL title game. The game, played in Green Bay City Stadium on New Year's Eve of 1961, gave the players, coaches and fans something extra to celebrate. "Hail to Title Town, Packers World Champions" screamed the *Milwaukee Sentinel* headline. Head Coach Lombardi proclaimed that "This is the greatest team in the history of the National Football League."

I have a vivid memory of that shellacking the Pack dished out to the Giants. The sun was shining, the temperature for New Year's Eve was moderate, and there was no wind. As my wife and I sat in our seats (Row 50 at the 35 yard line) my thoughts were: how did the Green Bay Packers get that much better than the Giants? I believe the Packers peaked during that game – that is, all subsequent victories would not occur with that degree of dominance.

The 1962 season

As had become their habit, the Packers won all six of their exhibition games as well as their first two season games. In their third game they trounced their archrivals, the Chicago Bears, 49-0. Coach Lombardi was said to have lost sleep over beating, by such a large margin, his colleague and friend, George Halas.

The fourth opponent for the Pack was the also undefeated Detroit Lions. Detroit led 7-6 with less than a minute left in the game. The Packers were the beneficiary of a bone-headed play by Detroit quarterback, Milt Plum, who threw a pass toward Terry Barr, but was intercepted by Herb Adderly on the Green Bay 45 yard line and returned to the Detroit 20. Green Bay moved the ball down to the 14, and then a Hornung field goal won the game 9-7 for the Packers. Following the gift from Lion quarterback, the Packers racked up six wins in a row to give them a 10-0 record. The six losers were the Bears again, the Colts twice, the 49ers, the Vikings and the Eagles. As payback for the 1960 title defeat by the Eagles, the Packers unloaded on them, gaining 628 yards and outscoring them 49-0.

The 10-0 Packers were preparing for their annual Thanksgiving Day visit – despised by Lombardi - to Detroit for a match with the Lions. This time the Packers were never in the game, primarily because of the overwhelming rush led by Detroit defensive tackles, Alex Karras and Roger Brown. The score at halftime was 23-0 in favor of Detroit and 26-0 at the end of three quarters. Finally, Green Bay scored two touchdowns despite Starr being sacked an unbelievable eleven times. The final score was 26-14.

The Packers were now 10-1, for a one game lead over the Lions. Both teams won the following week, leaving two games yet to be played by each team. The Lions defeated the second-year Vikings while the Packers traveled to San Francisco and got off to a poor start, 21-10 at half time. The Packers scored three touchdowns in the second half, held the 49ers scoreless and won going away 31-21 for a season record of 13-1 and another conference championship.

The title game was played in New York against the Giants in brutal weather conditions of 50 mph winds combined with a 15-degree temperature. The wind precluded any significant passing, and the frozen "slag" traumatized running back Jim Taylor each time he was tackled. Green Bay scored on a seven-yard slant run by Taylor and three Jerry Kramer field goals. The Green Bay defense lived up to its reputation by limiting the Giants to only one score, the return of a blocked punt for a touchdown. Final score was 16-7. Final 1962 records: Packers 14-1, Giants 12-3.

The 1963 season

The Packers opened the 1963 season with a loss to the College All-Star team, 20-17. Green Bay native, Ron VanderKelen, passed for a touchdown to fellow Wisconsin Badger teammate, Pat Richter, for one of their scores. Hornung and Lions defensive tackle Alex Karras had been suspended by NFL commissioner, Pete Rozelle, prior to the start of the season, for betting on NFL games. The loss of Hornung could have been greater but for the contribution of his replacement, Tom Moore.

The Packers lost their regular season opening game for the third time in the last four years, 10-3, to the hated Bears. A 3-3 halftime score was supplemented by a Bear touchdown following Taylor's fumble on the Packer 33. Four Starr interceptions and Taylor's puny 33 rushing yards contributed to the Packers' loss.

Recovering from the Bear loss, the Packers won eight games in a row, but not without a price. In the sixth game of the season (a 30-7 win over the Cardinals), Starr broke his right hand while falling awkwardly when he was running out of bounds. Keeping the injury a secret, Lombardi traded for Rams understudy Zeke Bratkowski, to complement the very little used quarterback, John Roach.

Roach won the last three of the eight-game winning streak. The now 8-1 Packers lost to the Bears 26-7 but beat the 49ers two days following the Kennedy assassination. Starr was back from his right hand injury for the Thanksgiving Day Detroit game that ended in a 13-13 tie. The Bears tied two of their final five games to finish 11-1-2, compared to the 11-2-1 Packers. In the NFL title game, the Bears beat the Giants 14-10 in eleven- degree Wrigley Field weather.

Bart Starr and Jim Taylor in the delivery room

Missing out on their attempt to win their third title in a row was frustrating to the Packers, especially their great quarterback, Bart Starr. Much of this frustration quickly dissipated for Starr, however, as he and his wife looked forward to the arrival of their second child, due in early February 1964.

Approximately two years before the Starr baby was due, Jimmy Taylor's wife Dixie (also my patient) had delivered their son Chip. Jimmy had petitioned me to be allowed in the delivery room to witness the birth. At that time Bellin Hospital had no policy permitting or excluding fathers from the delivery room. Also, prior to that time, deliveries often occurred with general anesthesia, which precluded any support a prospective father might provide to his wife during the delivery process. The nurses and I evaluated Jimmy's request, and since the rules relating to the spouse's presence during delivery were silent, Taylor, gowned and with a surgical cap and mask in place, was welcomed into the delivery room.

A little background information on Jimmy's philosophy as a Packer running back seems in order here. His preference, when faced by would-be tacklers, was to smash into them and knock them down - so they would remember him – rather than running around them. When Lombardi asked Taylor about his philosophy, he replied, "Coach, you can't make a greyhound out of a bulldog." In addition, Taylor thought that smashing into and running over the would-be tackler was the shortest route to the goal line.

Yet, despite his reputation as being the toughest running back in the NFL, Taylor fainted during the delivery, being let down to the delivery room floor gently by two nearby nurses. After a brief recovery, he couldn't wait to be helped out of the room by the same two nurses. Years later, Jimmy, Paul Hornung and Bart Starr returned to Green Bay to help celebrate the 2005 opening of the new Bellin Hospital lobby and tower, and I enjoyed reminiscing about his delivery room mishap.

As you might guess, I was accused of violating a non-existent delivery room rule about visitors for the Taylor delivery. The good news is that the "uproar" over my transgression led to the development of rules regarding the presence of spouses or significant others in the delivery room - if the delivery was to occur with local anesthesia, these visitors were allowed in. In that sense, the Taylors were pioneers and, it could be said, ran interference for the Starrs, prior to the February 1, 1964 birth of their second son, Brett Michael. By this time the delivery room policy had been solidly in place.

As indicated above, the Starrs put aside their frustration concerning the missed third Packer title, using the expected birth of their second son to put their lives in proper perspective. As Bart wrote, "The thrill of being with Cherry during the delivery and actually witnessing the miracle of birth, quickly put my life back into focus." Unlike Taylor, Bart did not faint, and in fact was cool throughout the delivery process.

Bart and Cherry Starr were and are the nicest couple one could ever meet. True to their form was a letter I received from Cherry on April 8, 1974 expressing appreciation for all that I had done for them:

4/8/74
Cherry Starr
Dear Herb,
Because you have been so attentive to my needs over the years, I simply want you to know how much I appreciate the exceptional professional care you have given me. You have never been too busy to return a phone call or see me on short notice, and that is comforting since I operate on a somewhat hectic schedule also.

You have shown much courage to speak out on issues that could damage you professionally, and I commend you for doing so.

Bart and I are proud to live in a community where people really do care for each other and are willing to extend themselves when special care is needed.

Thank you and God bless you for all you do for others.
Cherry

The 1964 season

The Packers rejoiced with the news that Commissioner Rozelle, believing that a one-year suspension was sufficient punishment for Hornung's sins, reinstated him in March of 1964.

The Packers beat the Bears in their opener 23-12, helped by Hornung's three field goals and 77 rushing yards. That was his one splash for the season. Following their Bear win, they lost three of the next five games, largely due to Hornung's missed field goals. Three games later, the Vikings blocked another Hornung PAT attempt. In the sixth game, the Packers again lost to the Colts 24 – 21, with Hornung missing four field goals. The common refrain around Green Bay at that time went like this: Question –"How's it going, Paul?" Answer, "I can't kick."

The Packers closed the season going 5-1-1 in the second half, finishing at 8-5-1 instead of the 11-2-1 record that could have been achieved with just an average kicker. The team outscored their opponents by almost 100 points (342-245).

Starr's play was better than that of any prior season, completing 163 of 272 passes (59.9%) for 2144 yards, 15 touchdowns and only four interceptions. In my view, it was Hornung, who single-handedly cost the Packers another championship by missing an incredible 26 out of 38 field goal attempts plus some extra points. What was Lombardi thinking by sticking with him for the entire season as the chances for another championship dwindled away? Was the great coach influenced by his personal fondness of Hornung?

The 1965 season

Approaching the 1965 season, Lombardi traded and drafted for better players, the most important of whom was Don Chandler from the Giants, who replaced Hornung as the place kicker. On September 11, 1965, City Stadium was renamed Lambeau Field in honor of Earl "Curly" Lambeau, the Packer founder, who had died the previous June.

The Packers opened their 1965 season with four straight victories, including wins over the Steelers, Colts, Bears and 49ers. At the half of their fifth game they were trailing Detroit 21-3. Lombardi inserted the recovering Jerry Kramer into the offensive line for the second half to better protect Starr from the brutal rush of Alex Karras. With Starr passing for three long touchdowns and the defense shutting down the Lions, the Packers won 31-21. With four games remaining, the Packers, at 8-2, trailed only the 8-1-1 Baltimore Colts. Unfortunately, the Packers lost to the Rams the following week.

In the next game, the Packers beat the Vikings while the Colts were not only upset by the Bears, but in addition, lost quarterback Johnny Unitus to injury for the rest of the season. With the Packers one half game ahead of the Colts, it was fitting that the Colts were the opponent for game 13. A couple of Packer wins would clinch another Western conference championship. With Hornung running for five touchdowns, the Packers prevailed 42-27. The season ended with a Packer tie against the 49ers combined with a Colt victory, resulting in identical 10-3-1 records for the two frontrunners. With two season victories over the Colts that year, the Packers were awarded home-field advantage, and the playoff game was scheduled for the newly named Lambeau Field.

The Colts were not only without their star quarterback, Johnny Unitus, but also his understudy, Gary Cuozzo, because of injuries. Hornung suffered an injury on the first play from scrimmage, and Starr suffered a broken rib from a hard block following an interception. Zeke Bratkowski came in for Starr, and Tom Matte, an option halfback, started at quarterback for the Colts. The Packers fell behind in the first half, 10-0, but in the second half Hornung pushed over the goal line following an errant Colt punt and later Chandler (thank God it was not Hornung) kicked a disputed field goal to tie the game. With the overtime extending to 13 minutes and 39 seconds, Chandler kicked another field goal to give the Packers an overtime victory.

Bring on the Browns, Eastern Conference champions, was the chant of the Packer fans. Five inches of snow had accumulated on the field by noon of the championship game, leaving Lambeau Field mushy and soft. A later rain turned the field into mud. At the start of the contest, Starr completed a few short passes to Taylor and Hornung prior to a long bomb to Carroll Dale for a touchdown. Taylor and Hornung got the ground game going, and the Packers pulled out a 23-12 win in the title game. It was amazing to see how Lombardi had maintained the quality of the team to allow the Pack to be in contention for the title year after year.

The 1966 season

The NFL merged with the American Football League (AFL) on June 8, 1966, setting the stage for the first-ever Super Bowl at the end of the season. All players were free agents at that time, so Lombardi had to shell out big bucks to sign Donny Anderson of Texas Tech and Jim Grabowski of Illinois to replace the injured Hornung and the worn-out

Taylor. The Packers cruised through the season, winning 12 and losing two by a measly total of four points. Starr was voted MVP by his fellow league players while completing 156 of 251 passes for 2257 yards. He threw 14 touchdowns with only three interceptions for a rating of 104.9. Meanwhile, the Packers returned six opponents' interceptions for touchdowns.

The 12-2 Packers were hosted by the 10-3-1 Dallas Cowboys for the title game, pitting the highest scoring team, Dallas (who scored 31.8 points per game), against the stingiest defense, the Packers (who allowed only 11.6 points per game). The Packers led 14-0 early but by only 21-17 at the half. In the end, they intercepted Dallas quarterback Don Meredith's pass in the end zone to salvage a 34-27 win.

Super Bowl I, January 15, 1967

In the first Super Bowl, the AFL Champion Kansas City Chiefs faced the NFL Champion Green Bay Packers. The Packers were a 13-point favorite in the game, which was to be played in the Los Angeles Memorial Coliseum. With the Chiefs out-gaining the Packers in yardage, 181-164, and in first downs, 11 to 9, and being behind at half time only 14-10, they were exuberant and believed they would win the game. However, the exuberance was premature, as Starr eventually completed 16 of 23 passes for 250 yards and two touchdowns. The Packers won easily, 35-10, with Starr claiming the MVP of the game as well as the League MVP. How much higher could he go?

The 1967 season

Paul Hornung was selected from the list posted by the Packers for the expansion team, the New Orleans Saints, and Taylor, who had played out his option the previous year, was signed by the same team, thus keeping the duo together.

The Packers opened the season by defeating the College All Stars, 27-0, and as usual won all of their exhibition games. However, during the pre-season Starr severely bruised his ribs, had a shoulder injury, and suffered a badly sprained right thumb, limiting his grasp on the football. But he handled adversity well and always seemed to have his priorities right. Packer Jerry Kramer, reporting on Starr's attendance at the First United Methodist Church in Green Bay, quoted Pastor Roger Bourland: "One of his (Starr's) greatest characteristics" said Bourland, impressed with the balance in Starr's life, "is that he does so much for people in a personal way with his time, talent and money and most of them do not know he is responsible." On the team, he took spiritual leadership. "He has been very influential in bringing many of the Packers to church services," Bourland explained. "Four and one half hours before each game, half an hour before breakfast, we get together and read from the Bible and say a few prayers and sometimes have a little discussion led by Bart and Carroll Dale," said Kramer. About 20 players regularly attended.

The Packers tied the Lions in their 1967 regular season opener, 17-17, with Starr being harassed all afternoon by Alex Karras and throwing four interceptions, one more than he had the entire 1966 season. It got worse the next week, but despite five more interceptions, the Packers defeated the Bears 13-10. The Packers then defeated the Atlanta Falcons 23-0, despite Starr being knocked out of the game, taking a hit in the right armpit that numbed his throwing arm. All of the next week, Starr depended upon pain medication to get through practice, and even with that, his throwing was not sharp.

With the season record at 3-1-1, the Packers, following a victory against the Lions, headed for Yankee stadium to play the Giants. Behind at half time, 14-10, the Starr-led Packers erupted for 38 points in the second half, winning going away, 48-21. Despite the 38 second-half points, Starr was still hurting and had to leave the game in the fourth quarter. The following week, with Starr still in pain, the Packers squeaked out a 31-23 victory over the St. Louis Cardinals. The Packers next lost a heart-breaker 13-10 at Baltimore the following week after a Colts-recovered on-side kick resulted in a game-winning Unitus touchdown pass. Following a 13-0 win over the 49ers, the Pack was 7-2-1, and with a 17-13 victory over the Bears improved to 8-2-1, clinching the newly formed Central Division title and heading for the playoffs. Winning one of their last three games, the Packers finished with a regular season record of 9-4-1 and were scheduled for a playoff game in Milwaukee against the 11-1-2 Rams. The Rams, showing little respect for the Packers, boasted that they had broken the Packers' magic as a result of their defeating the Packers in an earlier game 27-24. With Starr playing injured for most of the 1967 season, he was intercepted 17 times while throwing for only nine touchdowns, for a poor quarterback rating of 64.4.

On paper, the Packers-Rams match-up definitely did not favor the Packers, who were thought to be old and injured – a poor combination! With the Rams up 7-0 early in the game, Starr threw an interception, giving the Rams the ball on the Packer 10-yard line. The defense held, forcing a field goal attempt, which Packer linebacker Robinson stuffed.

A sixty-seven yard touchdown run by Travis Williams tied the score, 7-7. A touchdown pass to Dale gave the Packers their first lead, 14-7, at the half. The Rams were held scoreless by the great Packer defense – especially that of Henry Jordan and Ray Nitschke – in the second half, with the Packers winning 28-7.

The Legendary Ice Bowl, December 31, 1967

With the coldest game in the history of the National Football League looming, Lombardi allowed his players to wear long underwear but not gloves for anyone except the linemen. Dave Robinson, an African American, jokingly asked for brown gloves to fool the Cowboys and Lombardi. A full house of 50,861 fans, wearing a wide variety of warm clothing, was in the stands, some more than two hours before kickoff. My wife and I chose sleeping bags for our outermost layer of clothing. The thing I remember best is the warm air emanating from the lungs of 50,000-plus fans with the formation of a misty fog blanketing the stands.

By game time the temperature was minus 13 degrees with a 5 mile per hour wind, putting the wind chill at minus 38 degrees. A pass to Boyd Dowler and another to Carroll Dale gave the Packers 14 points in the first half. Meanwhile, the Cowboys, profiting from two Green Bay fumbles, had ten points.

The third quarter was scoreless. The officials could not use their frozen whistles. Early in the fourth quarter, Dan Reeves threw an option pass for a 50-yard score, putting the Cowboys out front 17 – 14. The drama heightened with 4:50 left in the game when the Packers, with one chance left, had the ball on their own 32, 68 yards from victory. Starr first dumped the ball off to running back Donny Anderson. Chuck Mercein then gained seven yards, and Starr passed to Dowler for 13 more, getting the Packers to the Dallas 42. Anderson lost nine yards on an attempted end sweep, bringing the Pack back to their own 49-yard line. Starr, always calm, cool and collected, dumped passes off to Anderson for gains of twelve and nine yards, converting a first down with two yards more than needed!

With two minutes left, the ball was on the Dallas 30, and the Packers had a first down. Starr connected with Mercein for a 19-yard gain down the left side of the field where he was pushed out of bounds at the eleven. Mercein then ran for eight more yards, his progress impeded only when he ran into teammate Forest Gregg at the three-yard line. Anderson then gained one yard for a first down but had no gain on the following play. After a Green Bay timeout, Anderson, slipping and almost fumbling, was stopped again for no gain. With third down and

16 seconds left, the Packers called for their final timeout. Without telling anyone on the Green Bay team, Starr called his own number and sneaked over a Jerry Kramer block and in for the touchdown, giving the Packers the VICTORY, 20-17! After having seen Anderson slipping on the two previous plays, Starr held the same concern for Mercein, who all the Packers expected to carry the ball. Again it was a hot time in Green Bay for a New Year celebration.

The second Super Bowl game, January 14, 1968

The Oakland Raiders had won the AFL's Western division with a 13-1 record and then trounced Houston 41-7 for the league title. Super Bowl II was played in Miami's Orange Bowl before a sell-out crowd of 75,546. In preparation for the game, Lombardi told the players how proud he was of them, especially since, for the first time in the history of the National Football League, a team could win three successive league championships. Following other inspiring remarks, the team took to the field.

The Packers scored two early field goals followed by a 62-yard touchdown pass to Dowler for a 13-0 lead. The Raiders scored their only touchdown in the first half, giving the Packers a 16-7 halftime lead. The Packers took control of the game in the third quarter, scoring a touchdown and Chandler's third field goal for a 23-7 lead. In the fourth quarter Chandler kicked his fourth field goal, and Herb Adderly returned an interception 60 yards for a touchdown for a final score of 33-14.

Starr completed 13 of 24 passes for 202 yards with no interceptions and, for the second year in a row, was named the game's MVP.

Lombardi resigned as coach on February 1, 1968 but continued as General Manager for one year. He then became coach of the Washington Redskins, where he was at the time of his death on September 3, 1970.

Thus was the end of The Glory Years!!!

When we moved to Green Bay in 1959 the population was only 50,000, and it was unusual for a small town to have a professional sports team. Furthermore, it was the only community-owned team in the NFL and as I mentioned earlier, was one of the two remaining founding teams of the NFL, the other being the Chicago Bears.

The success of the Packers in the Glory Years made me an avid fan for life, taking much pride on their winning and pretending, as a Green Bay citizen, that I was partly responsible for their success. Whenever I traveled out of Wisconsin for attendance at medical meetings, I was recognized by one and all as "that guy from Green Bay." If I had been from Sheboygan, no one would have recognized or remembered me.

The Green Bay Packer mystique spread world-wide. While traveling in Japan, Dr. Edelblute, a Green Bay radiologist, mailed a post card addressed only to "the world's greatest quarterback," with absolutely no other address, and it was delivered to the Starr's home, whereupon Cherry quipped to Bart that it must have mistakenly arrived at their house and was really meant for Johnny Unitus! Green Bay citizens, at times, were ridiculed by the national press as being unsophisticated cheese heads who attended Packer games in hunting clothes. No one seemed to mind. Perhaps it was like the politician who cared not what they wrote about him as long as they spelled his name correctly.

Tail-gating usually began about two and one-half hours prior to kick-off, often with very elaborate grills and other equipment to prepare the famous beer and brat meal. We did not participate in tail-gating since we had a reserved parking space and would avoid heavy traffic by arriving just prior to the kick-off.

The community profited from all of the money funneled into town on home-game weekends as 72,000 fans, most of who were from out of town, descended upon Green Bay. In particular, the hotels, restaurants and gasoline stations were very busy, including some as far away as Appleton. Also Lambeau Field is used year-round by many organizations, further bolstering the Green Bay economy. Additional revenue comes from the sale of Packer paraphernalia – everything from foam cheeseheads to green and gold jerseys - in the Packer gift shop. Proceeds from Packer sales are routinely tops in the NFL.

When television announcers come to broadcast a game in Green Bay, they often speak of Lambeau Field, with its rich history, as the "frozen tundra," the hallowed ground of the famous Ice Bowl and home to many memorable games and players. Former NFL players from other teams often say that there was something truly special about coming to play at Lambeau Field. Some of the team's "legendary" status is thanks to the legend that was Vince Lombardi, winning coach of the first two Super Bowls for whom the Super Bowl trophy has been named ever since. Green Bay doesn't have the glamour and glitz of New York, Los Angeles, or other cities with NFL teams, but it has, nonetheless, taken on an iconic status in pages of American sports history. And there is nothing mysterious about the frenetic support the Packers enjoy from the local community and fans ("fanatics") around the state of Wisconsin. After all, it is in the team's charter that it will always be community-owned and can never be sold – a stipulation almost unheard of in professional sports. An independent observer might even conclude that what is most intriguing about the Packers is not whether they win or lose, but rather their amazing ability to bring a group of supporters together with a shared sense of belonging and purpose – it really is a social phenomenon.

On a sobering note, football, like boxing, is a violent game that results in major injuries to sometimes more than a third of a team's 53-man squad. Concussions seem to be increasing despite rule changes designed to reduce injuries. The Packers own star quarterback, Aaron Rodgers, suffered two concussions during the teams victory run this year to the Super Bowl. So why does a physician whose life's work has been devoted to enhancing human health, watch and enjoy this violent game - football - so much, yet not support boxing? I do not know the answer to that question. Selective morality, perhaps? An excuse I could use is the boost to the Green Bay economy "kicked off" with each home game. Whatever the reason, to live in Green Bay is to be a Green Bay Packer devotee, and I am no exception.

CHAPTER 7

/More research

WHILE THE PACKERS provided a welcome weekend respite, my thoughts quickly turned to my work as the sound of the Sunday crowd grew faint. In the fall of 1960, the presentation/publication bug bit me again, this time involving "The prevention and treatment of postpartum hemorrhage" which I presented at the ACOG District VI meeting in Chicago (November 11, 1960) and published in the February 1961 issue of the *Wisconsin Medical Journal*. Further presentations and publications occurring during that time period included the "Treatment of the incompetent cervix to prevent second trimester abortions," in the October 1962 issue of the *Wisconsin Medical Journal*.

"Paracervical block anesthesia in obstetrics," which I published in the March 7, 1964 issue of the *Journal of the American Medical Association*, was also presented at the annual meeting of the Wisconsin Society of Obstetrics and Gynecology in Racine, Wisconsin in October of 1962.

My next presentation was "Curettage as an office procedure," given at the annual meeting of District VI, in Milwaukee on November 23, 1963, the day after President Kennedy was assassinated. It was subsequently published in the July 1964 *Journal of Obstetrics and Gynecology*.

In October of 1965, I presented "Amniocentesis on Rh-sensitized women" at the annual meeting of the Wisconsin Society of Obstetricians and Gynecologists in Madison, Wisconsin. This was a part of a day-long program entitled "Rh problems and the sensitized mother." Amniocentesis involves drawing off some of the amniotic fluid that surrounds the fetus and subjecting it to spectrophotometric analysis for antibodies that could be harmful to the fetus by causing severe anemia. The four other speakers were full professors from prominent medical schools, and there I was without any faculty appointment. Two of the four speakers were from the two Wisconsin medical schools, one was from Boston, and one was from Winnipeg, Canada. Nevertheless, I believe that, at that time, my presentation was a very important contribution to the program, and I have no idea why I did not submit it for publication.

I remember that one of my Rh-sensitized study patients was pregnant with twins, which required the drawing off of the fluid from each of the separate twin sacs. I injected some dye into the first sac at the conclusion of drawing off the fluid. I then tapped the second sac and drew off clear fluid (no dye present), thus proving that I had not tapped the same sac twice.

On another front, my continued work as a member of the Maternal Mortality Study Committee helped me see the need for an article describing the latest recommendations for the management of Rh-negative patients. The Rh factor article was printed in the February 1975 edition of the *Wisconsin Medical Journal*. This article focused on the newer tests to improve the management and outcome for those pregnant women who were Rh-sensitized.

CHAPTER 8

Fear of flying

IN THE SUMMER of 1963 I was inducted into the American College of Surgeons at its annual meeting in San Francisco. We were joined by Dr. and Mrs. Kenneth Forbes on our train trip to attend the meeting. Following the two-day journey, during which time we were privileged to appreciate the beautiful scenery, especially the Colorado mountain area, we arrived in San Francisco. I do not remember much about the meeting except for two experiences: 1) the wife of a general practitioner who seemed to have a disproportionate number of patients "needing" surgery visited with us momentarily and then declared she needed to "circulate." The reception hall was filled with an estimated 3,000 to 5,000 physicians and their spouses. As a young physician, that was the first time I had an awareness of "social climbing." 2) the San Francisco trip was equally important because of my discovering a way to prevent my horrible fear of flying. After boarding the plane for the trip back to Green Bay, there was, as often happens, about a 45-minute delay due to some mechanical or luggage problem. To pacify us the flight attendant passed out large glasses of champagne with no limits on refills. By the time we took off an hour later, I was, for the first time in my life, the bravest passenger on the plane. I almost believed I could fly home without the benefit of the plane! Thereafter I used this fear-prevention measure of having one or two martinis before boarding the plane, – even before breakfast. By the early 1970s, with more experience flying, I no longer needed to do this.

In May of 1959, six weeks before I completed my residency, I decided to attend the ACOG Annual Clinical meeting in Atlantic City, New Jersey. Crystal and I, with our children, drove to Meadville, Pennsylvania and stayed a couple days with Crystal's brother Kenneth, who at that time was a professor in the Economics Department at Alleghany College, and his wife Audrey.

I had arranged for Dr. Bill Goddard, Iowa faculty member, to pick me up in his very small plane in Meadville for the rest of the trip to Atlantic City. This plan had many important pitfalls which I had not accounted for: 1) the actual size of his plane; 2) the height of Pennsylvania's mountains; 3) the effect of flying over mountains with the tremendous down drafts and 4) the level of my fear of flying.

After we safely landed in Atlantic City, I began to immediately plan for my return trip, which did not include getting into a plane, small or large. I ran into the late Dr. Lee Stevenson from Detroit and bummed a ride with him to Meadville in his Volkswagen Bug. And even though the mountains were still there and we careened down them at speeds I considered unsafe, I arrived back in Meadville scared but safe. Sweetie's first question on my return was, "How was your trip?" In describing my trip to others I claimed that I flew both ways.

In 1984 I was assisting John Menn, Appleton attorney, with the defense of an Ashland, Wisconsin obstetrician who had been sued, the plaintiff alleging he had failed to prevent cerebral palsy. In preparation for my Monday testimony, Attorney Menn and I flew to Superior, Wisconsin, near Ashland, Sunday afternoon in his private plane.

As soon as we started down the runway for take-off, I realized I had made a horrible mistake in flying with this 72-year old pilot with no co-pilot. Sitting next to him in the co-pilot's seat, I immediately watched every move Attorney Menn made as we took off as well as during the flight, and especially during our landing. I tried to disguise my fear by not asking an overwhelming number of questions but did want to know what I should know if I had to land the airplane.

After our landing in Superior I was immediately relieved of my fears until I realized we would be flying back to Appleton under a similar arrangement. Therefore, my anxiety continued during my testimony (we won the case anyway) and until I set my feet on the good earth following our return to Appleton.

CHAPTER 9

Helping out at the University of Wisconsin at Green Bay (UWGB)

IN THE EARLY 1960s, I began giving community lectures at the old "Cardboard Tech" rooms on Deckner Avenue, a forerunner of the University of Wisconsin-Green Bay (UWGB). Most of these lectures, which I continued to do until 1986, involved birth control methods, other women's rights issues, and the problems of over population. UWGB became a four-year, degree granting university in 1966, with a special emphasis on environmental concerns. Consistent with that focus, the university sponsored two conferences, in 1970 and 1971, involving Population Growth and Family Planning Programs. I chaired the Saturday morning session for the 1971 program.

In 1970, I started giving lectures in UWGB Professor John Shier's Population Dynamics 101 class. These lectures went beyond birth control methods and included a discussion of problems associated with over population: pollution of the environment, poverty, hunger, acceleration of the use of natural resources, and various social problems. While it is hard to tell exactly how much impact I had as a guest lecturer, feedback from one particular student made me believe that I was on the right track:

> *December 6, 1970*
> *Dear Dr. Sandmire,*
> *I am a student at UWGB taking the Population Dynamics course.*
> *As a guest lecturer, you are not able to receive much feedback from the students as to how you are coming across, and that is why I am writing.*

I think you are doing a wonderful job. Your subject matter is something we all should be aware of and understand and yet few of us did before this course. You know and understand your subject so well that you don't refer to your notes. It gives us the feeling that you are talking to us and not at us.

I am also impressed that a doctor would take time from his practice to come talk to us. This makes me see that you are personally concerned about the population problem and about us as individuals and our "population problems."

I have enjoyed your lectures. Thank you.

Mary Howard

Although I do not remember for certain, I assume that it was after reading her letter that I probably volunteered to continue teaching for a long, long time, lecturing for Professor Shier as well as for Drs. Thea and Paul Sager, both professors in UWGB's College of Human Biology. The following letter from Thea Sager also provided important feedback information:

University of Wisconsin- Green Bay
July 9, 1981
Dr. Herbert Sandmire
704 South Webster
Green Bay, WI 54301
Dear Herb:
I feel that whatever I say will not be adequate and cannot really express how much I appreciate your willingness, each year, to participate as extensively as you do in the "Fertility, Reproduction and Family Planning" course. Your lectures are interesting, informative, thought-provoking, and well-presented. My hope is that in the future, students will continue to benefit from your presence in the classroom.
Sincerely,
Thea Sager, Ph.D.
College of Human Biology

About this time, because of my publications, Dr. Keettel issued the first of several invitations for me to join the OB/Gyn Department at the University of Iowa where he was Chairperson. Feeling as I did that research activities could be conducted while in private practice and also that long-term follow up of research subjects was more available to researchers in private practice compared to those in an academic setting, I remained in Green Bay.

CHAPTER 10

Vacations: Mid 60s to mid 70s

OUR VACATION DESTINATIONS from the mid-1960s to the mid-1970s involved camping out at our children's "rich" Uncle Ty's Tuck-A-Way Farm and campground. When our son David was in third grade, his class was given an assignment to write their family history. David wrote that he had a rich uncle – turned out to be my brother, Uncle Ty, who owned and operated a farm together with a campground on his property. The combination of many riding horses and a team of Clydesdales denoted richness to David. Ty was pleasantly surprised when he found out that he was "rich."

Also, during that same time period, in July, we would share our vacations at Strege's cottages in Ephraim, Wisconsin with either the Sherwood or Steinbrink families. The children enjoyed, among other things, walking to Wilson's store for ice cream and taffy. In July of 1967, we journeyed with the Philipp family to Expo 67 in Montreal, camping along our way through Canada. Unfortunately, Kevin became stomach sick on the way, which gave me a chance to use my medical training – by the expertly timed placing of a pan, to catch the vomit which was about to be released from Kevin in the upper bunk.

Winter vacations involved traveling to the Wisconsin-Michigan border to King's Gateway Inn, often with the Johnstons or the Ottums. Activities included ice skating, snowmobiling, swimming in the indoor pool, and bowling. One weekend at King's Gateway, the temperature dropped to 30 degrees below zero. Paying attention to the weather forecast, I took the car battery into the resort and set it on top of the radiator. The next day, while everyone else was having their battery boosted by a service truck, I returned our battery to the car and promptly started the motor with no booster service cost. This proves what I suspected; a warm battery has more power than a cold one.

Although coaching and attendance at Little League baseball games would not generally be described as being on vacation, it did provide a time when our whole family could share a common interest and spend time together. Our Little League experience began in 1966 when our oldest son, Kevin, was ten years old. At that time I became the assistant manager of the Allouez Orioles. Our manager was ecstatic over the draft picks we made that year. Personally, I, in silence, wondered if we were truly lucky or if our draft picks just did not impress the other seven managers.

I was "promoted" to manager in our second Little League year. As manager I could instill our philosophy of playing hard but fair, having respect for other team members and their coaches, and being polite to everyone. These same principles applied to me and my coaching staff. Interacting with young kids in this venue was a welcome break from my professional life. Our players came in all shapes and sizes, and no two were alike. Some exuded extreme confidence while others approached the game with considerable trepidation. I remember a young boy named Timmy who always needed to go to the bathroom when it was his turn at bat. As expected, we had to deal with the occasional overly aggressive parent; however, they were the exception, probably because the parents had respect for the fact that a busy physician would take the time to coach a Little League team.

Game day was exciting for Sweetie and me and all of our children. Sweetie would bring the bats, balls, the catcher's mask and chest protector as well as all of our kids, and I would come to the park directly from work. The girls, Cheryl and Yvonne, and the younger boys, too young for Little League, enjoyed functioning as cheerleaders. For me, it was a time of bonding with my whole family as well as doing something worthwhile for the community. I was "killing two birds with one stone" as could be said.

On occasion, my own sons led the team to victories. The Thursday, May 30, 1974 *Green Bay Press Gazette* reported that "The Sandmire brother act boosted the Orioles to an 11-2 win over the Cubs in the Allouez Little League. Dave Sandmire cracked a home run and Mike Sandmire was the winning pitcher in the season opener." We teased 10-year old Dave that he must have closed his eyes and swung, and that the ball must have hit a jet stream to make it over the fence (it was his only home run in Little League).

Following each season we had an Allouez Orioles picnic to reward all of the players and to say good-by to our twelve-year olds.

Our Orioles were league champions for 1972 and 1973 and the team presented me with a trophy inscribed, "To the greatest coaching staff in the world, Thanks, the Orioles – 1975."

Little Leaguers are aged 10 to 12, so as each of our sons turned thirteen, they transitioned from players to members of my coaching staff. In addition to our regular work with the Orioles, my son Kevin and I also managed the Allouez All-stars from 1975 to 1978, which often involved travel to other cities.

Over the past 44 years, people have occasionally come up to me to ask if I remembered them as an Oriole Little League player. The last time that happened was in 2007 in a Maui Sports bar, while we were watching the Green Bay Packers play. To my surprise, a middle-aged man addressed me as "Coach." It was Johnny Effland, who played for me 33 years earlier.

Over all, the time spent with the Allouez Orioles was a very rewarding experience. I cannot think of a better activity I could have been involved in for those 13 years.

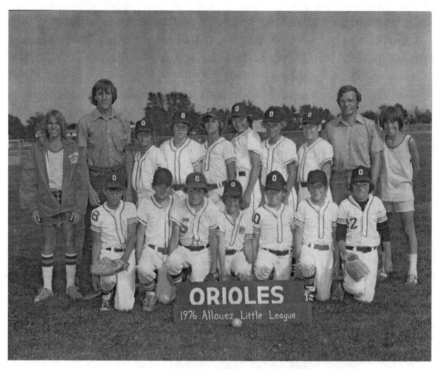

The League Championship Allouez Orioles with
four Sandmire coaches (1976)

CHAPTER 11

Beaumont Clinic / UW Preceptor

HAVING SUCCESSFULLY RECRUITED four pediatricians, two internists, and two general surgeons, Dr. Austin and I opened the Beaumont Clinic on Webster Avenue in Allouez, Wisconsin. Six months later, a third obstetrician, Dr. John Utrie, joined the clinic. One might question my motivation for starting a multi-specialty clinic after rejecting two offers from clinics during the process of selecting an area for my practice. The reason for the change in my philosophy was the desire, for the convenience of our patients, to have access to inter-specialty consultation and laboratory and x-ray service all "under one roof." 1965 was the year of the inauguration of Medicare and Medicaid, programs that were very helpful to low-income individuals and also immediately resulted in more patients in our office. As we got busier, the only "bump in the road" that first year was that the administrator we had hired was unable to "cut the mustard" and was terminated at the end of the year. I was appointed as merely an "interim" administrator, but as it turned out, I continued in that capacity for the next six years.

As a University of Wisconsin Medical School preceptor

During the very early 1960s Dr. Austin and I began to give lectures to the Bellin School of Nursing students. Covering all of the major topics within our specialty, we provided lectures for 12 hours of each quarter. This continued until the early 1980s at which time the nursing faculty developed taped lectures for similar purposes. This was my first teaching assignment for the time period after we came to Green Bay in 1959, and it foreshadowed my involvement in the University of Wisconsin Medical School's preceptorship program.

The preceptorship program at the University of Wisconsin began in 1926, the same year the medical school increased from a two-year to a four-year curriculum. This innovative program was an historic first and was subsequently duplicated by medical schools across the United States. It entailed the placement of medical students under the direction of local physicians, in their community, for eight to thirteen weeks of the students' senior year of medical school. This represented a partial return to the physician-apprentice medical education model in operation until the late 1800s.

Initially, almost all of the programs in Wisconsin began with the preceptee (senior medical student) residing in the preceptor's home. Beginning in the late 1940s, arrangements were made for the student to receive room and board at the local hospital. The program provided the student an opportunity to observe and participate in the practice of medicine in the "real world." In addition to learning how to treat patients in the local community, the student was able to observe how the physician interacted with local citizens, service clubs, public school systems, and local governmental officials. It must be remembered that in the 1930s and 1940s the physician was one of only a few citizens whose education extended beyond high school.

The students were able to observe the lifestyle of their teachers in the local community: how did the preceptor balance the competing responsibilities to patients, spouse, and family? Was the physician a good spouse and parent? Did the doctor have a good relationship with his or her children? Were vacations part of the physician's life, and if so, how was coverage arranged to meet the needs of the physician's patients? How did the doctor interact with patients calling after office hours? Which patient concerns needed immediate attention and which could be addressed in the office the following day? These were all questions that the preceptorship was designed to answer. If the patients concerns required attention before the next day, the preceptee would accompany the preceptor at all hours and observe the management of the patient's condition, accomplished by either a house call or an emergency room visit. The preceptor and the family both profited from having live-in, goal-oriented, medical students who served as role models for the children in the preceptor's family.

I was asked to become one of the 20 preceptors (my first faculty appointment) in the spring of 1966. I accepted and continued in that capacity until 1986. Our first preceptee was Howard Johnson. As ours was an obstetrics and gynecology practice, it was natural that the Green Bay preceptor program would be selected by those senior students who had already chosen Ob/Gyn for their career. If students didn't fit into that category, I assigned them to other specialty and family medicine physicians. Students also gained experience in the emergency room on nights and weekends, an integral part of the Green Bay preceptorship program. The preceptees were provided with housing in the old part of St. Vincent Hospital, formerly the nun's quarters, and were also provided a meal pass for use in the St. Vincent Hospital cafeteria.

Toward the end of Howard Johnson's preceptorship, Sarah Alden, a *Green Bay Press Gazette* reporter, captured the goals we had set for the Green Bay preceptorship program in an insightful article:

The young doctor gains confidence
Medical students find the preceptorship program offers a chance to apply their knowledge, and it aids their mentors
By Sarah Alden, Press Gazette staff writer

Somewhere between a lecture on anatomy and an office full of patients, a physician must gain confidence that he not only knows the medicine he studied in textbooks, but can practice it with deft fingers and an eye for each person's illness.

For the first time a University of Wisconsin Medical School student - Howard Johnson of Sturgeon Bay – is acquiring some of that confidence in Green Bay, under the supervision of local physicians.

A Green Bay physician, Dr. Herbert F. Sandmire, and Green Bay medical facilities, including Beaumont Clinic and St. Vincent Hospital emergency ward, were approved by the university this year to participate in the "preceptorship" program.

Under the preceptorship, founded in Wisconsin in 1926 and now popular in many states, a senior medical student spends 13 weeks under the guidance of one or several community physicians.

Dr. Sandmire, an obstetrician on the Beaumont Clinic staff, is Johnson's preceptor and responsible for his experience here.

Johnson, son of Mr. and Mrs. Herbert Johnson of Sturgeon Bay, has spent 3 weeks with an obstetrician, caring for mothers; six weeks with internists and surgeons and is now starting his three weeks with a pediatrician.

He has a room in St. Vincent Hospital, he also eats in the cafeteria. The arrangement enables him to be on call on nights and weekends to learn emergency ward procedures, another requirement of the preceptorship.

Both Dr. Sandmire and his temporary protégé are expressive about the benefits they've already witnessed.

Dr. Sandmire pointed out that "University hospital wards do not represent a cross-section of community patients."

Or as Johnson puts it, "Without the preceptorship, it would be possible to graduate from medical school without ever seeing the measles or sewing up a laceration."

They explain that University patients often are physician referrals from throughout the state and have complicated diseases. Others are welfare or student health cases.

"We don't see many of the acute problems or accident cases common to a community," Johnson pointed out.

He has been impressed with local physicians' approach to this vital portion of his education. "They include me in what they do, without expecting me to take up their own specialties." He explained this would confuse most medical students at his stage, because he and most of his classmates have not decided what specific aspect of medicine to pursue.

And the internship still ahead of them is standard under Wisconsin law.

"It is marvelous to learn this way. Of course there's a gradual assumption of medical skills. But the confidence you gain from seeing and then doing (with supervision) is something."

"For example, I've read all about the process of the infant coming through the birth canal, but that's not like really delivering a baby."

He said he knows how heart disease should be treated - basically, "but here I can see how 20 doctors treat it with personal variations and I can decide how I am best at doing it. I get a broader scope."

Sandmire emphasized that the preceptorship gives students a chance to observe and evaluate the social, economic and environmental factors bearing upon a disease and its management.

Patients in the university hospital are out of their surroundings, he explained. Here patients are in their environment.

"A patient's problem may be interesting scientifically, but you must never lose sight of the individual, with his apprehension and his particular personality," the obstetrician said.

"That's true," Johnson echoed. "I've even found out no two wounds are alike."

He learned that in the emergency ward. "I'd had experience helping a Duluth, Minn., plastic surgeon and I thought I knew suturing pretty well. Yet these general practitioners – not plastic surgeons – have shown me many new things, and how much they know."

"One of them usually calls," he laughed at the remembrance, "Come here, Howard. There's something I want to teach you – right now!" And it's usually worth his running.

He said he especially wanted to thank physicians Grondall, Wesley McNeal, Richard Jensen, and Gerald Merline in addition to Wallace MacMullen for their interest.

One night a little girl had a cut tongue "and I didn't know how to sew up a tongue."

At another time, in a quite normal delivery, the obstetrician showed him what to do "when we had momentary difficulty getting the baby's shoulders out. When a baby's coming, you can't run and look it up. You've got about three minutes."

Johnson has been pleased that so many Green Bay patients have understood what he likes to call "the spirit of medical education," at least after the physician's explanation.

Dr. Sandmire had to explain it in more detail to one woman.

"Medical education involves problems different from most other kinds of education," he said. "There is no substitute for experience with real, individual patients. Every doctor who graduates must have it."

"If we are deficient as teachers, or do not participate, the future patients of the future doctors will be the only ones to suffer. To the extent that we are successful, they will benefit."

That woman accepted that, because she could see herself in the position of the future patient.

"And I'd like to think no matter what neophytes we are, we medical students can do good for patients," Johnson said. He illustrated by noting the patient histories done in depth by medical students during their four years are the university hospital's most complete records. "Because we were learning, we had to take down everything to learn the routine approach."

Dr. Sandmire said people might wonder why physicians would be so willing to participate in so time-consuming program. "But teaching is the best way to learn. The student provides an added incentive for keeping abreast of modern medicine."

Just as the student has to practice, the physician has to keep reading the medical journals, he emphasized.

As Dr. Sandmire sees it, "If we were to get 10 years behind, these new graduates would be the first to know it."

The Green Bay preceptorship program continued in a normal, unabated fashion until the mid-to late-1970s, at which time the students were expelled from their housing at St. Vincent Hospital. The reason, as explained by hospital personnel, was that the medical students were causing a "rumpus" in their quarters. When I interviewed the medical students for their explanation of their expulsion, they provided the following information: 1. they had also heard the periodic "rumpus," 2. they were determined, because of the possibility of being blamed, to find out the true cause of the noise, and 3. they discovered the "rumpus" noise to be emanating from a hormonal encounter between a nurse anesthetist (call room in the same area) and a surgeon. The dilemma: what should be done with the information discovered by the students through their detective work. In the end, the students said nothing (nor did I), and they started to reside in our home, as they would for the next eight years, two to five students at a time.

As mentioned, the preceptorship program is exceedingly and mutually beneficial to the student as well as to the preceptor and his or her family. Therefore, the expulsion was not a disappointment to us as we could see the students being role models for our two younger sons who were still at home. St. Vincent Hospital continued to sponsor the meal pass and all other benefits for the program.

The Green Bay preceptorship was exceedingly popular, testimony to the excellent teaching abilities of the Green Bay physicians and hospital personnel. Indeed, their willingness to teach is exemplified by the fact that in my 20 years of experience with the program, I never experienced a turn-down when asking a Green Bay physician to share his or her patients with a senior medical student. During this period, more than 200 medical students were enrolled in the Green Bay program.

The following is one student's expression of appreciation for the Green Bay preceptorship learning experience. Notice his signature, "Med. IV," followed by the "Professor," my nickname for all of my students:

7 October 1987
Herbert F. Sandmire, M. D.
OB-GYN Associates of Green Bay, Ltd.
704 South Webster Avenue
Green Bay, WI 54301

Dear Dr. Sandmire,
First, let me thank you for an enjoyable month of learning. Not only did I gain a greater knowledge of obstetrics and gynecology, but I was made aware of issues concerning physicians and society.

Second, please extend my thanks to those who were of help to me while I was with you – the nurses at St. Vincent's and Bellin, your office staff, Dr. Bechtel, Dr. DeMott, the residents, and the emergency personnel.

Third, I am enclosing a brochure about the Women's Health Center in Madison. I hope that it is of aid to you.

Once again, my deepest thanks to you for sharing your knowledge and insight. I can say without reservation that my month with you was one of the best learning experiences that I have had while in medical school.

Respectfully,
Jerry J. Miller, MED IV
The "Professor"

In 1980, our on-the-job training expanded to include family practice residents as well. I was asked by the University of Wisconsin Medical School at Madison to set up and become the director of the Green Bay rotation for advanced obstetrics. Originally, this was to be used by the Madison Family Medicine residency program for improvement of their residency's obstetrical experience. The initial program was also available to the University of Wisconsin Family Medicine programs in Eau Claire, Wausau and Appleton. Soon thereafter we accepted family medicine residents from other programs in the United States and Canada.

Our clinical teaching expanded still further in 1985 to include family practice physicians enrolled in our obstetrics mini-fellowship program. Being over-extended in teaching responsibilities, I relinquished the preceptorship program in 1986.

CHAPTER 12

Paul Ehrlich / Environment / ZPG

THE PUBLICATION OF Paul Ehrlich's book, *the Population Bomb*, raised an awareness of the dangers of over-population for many of us. Particularly worrisome was the world population doubling time of 37 years at the time of release of Ehrlich's book in 1968. Doubling time for countries varied from every 20 years in the Philippines to every 175 years for Austria and 63 years for the U.S. Ehrlich exposed the expanded use of natural resources which population growth engendered as well as its adverse effect on our environment - all prior to a time when global warming was even a concern. Considering all of the other concerns in 1968, Ehrlich's warnings mostly fell on deaf ears. Is it again time to push for population stabilization as we did forty years ago? Imagine the problems we will face if there is another doubling of the U.S. and world population (hunger, pollution, global warming and social unrest).

Actually, at the risk of sounding preachy, I have observed that the average U.S. citizen either seems to not know or not care about environmental concerns. The evidence for this can be seen on any highway as drivers routinely travel 70 to 75 miles per hour in over-sized vehicles. During World War II, the speed limit was 35 mph because driving at that speed maximized fuel efficiency. Today's drivers sacrifice 15% of the fuel efficiency available at 55 mph and another 40-45% by driving large gas guzzling automobiles.

Congress contributes to the wasteful usage of gasoline by not taxing it, as they do in Europe to a cost double that in the U.S. Higher taxes and costs for gasoline will reduce the usage significantly – as already proven during the few times gasoline has exceeded four dollars per gallon in the U.S. If the higher gas tax presented a hardship on the citizens, taxes on other things such as income could be reduced by a like amount. When will we see this idea put into our tax laws? Cannot those in Congress see the advantages of this common-sense, win–win solution? Individuals would use less gasoline and cause less pollution while still having the same or more after-tax income (more if they drove less). Likewise, most people do not open the windows in the summer-time to get the cooling effect of the night-time temperature. In our home, the tolerable temperature is anything between 67 and 78 degrees. It is remarkable how these measures can reduce the energy cost associated with obtaining comfortable temperatures. I recommend that everyone try them to demonstrate for themselves how they can save on energy costs, be comfortable, and at the same time be friendly to our environment. In addition we need to speed up our conversion to solar and wind energy use.

Paul Ehrlich reported that half of the world's population was under-nourished, five million children in India were starving each year, and only three countries in the entire world were significant exporters of food: the United States, Canada, and Australia.

In 1973, at the time of the first Arab oil embargo, we replaced our two medium-sized automobiles (one a station wagon) with one small Ford Pinto, and I began to ride my bike three and one half miles to work on a daily basis, which was beneficial to both my internal and everyone else's external environment. As an educated person, I have also felt the responsibility to set an example for others in our office building who should be concerned for our environment. Sadly, up to my last day of work, thirty- seven years later, no one, to my knowledge, has followed my bike-riding example.

In 1995 my wife's 13-year old Renault Encore died on her during a trip back to Green Bay from Shawano. She called her brother who brought her home. She donated her car to Rawhide, a charitable organization affiliated with Bart and Cherry Starr. They provide a home for wayward boys who get experience repairing automobiles.

I suspected, but she never admitted, that she was happy that her car finally broke down. She shopped, with considerable enthusiasm, for another car, ultimately arriving home with a new Honda Civic that, at $13,000, was well within our budget.

About two years later she got rear-ended while stopped at an intersection, the car suffering a small, rear-end dent and slight loosening of the rear panels. We had the damaged car assessed by three automobile repair shops. The lowest bid came in at $1700. Since the damages sustained did not interfere with the operation or safety of the car, we asked

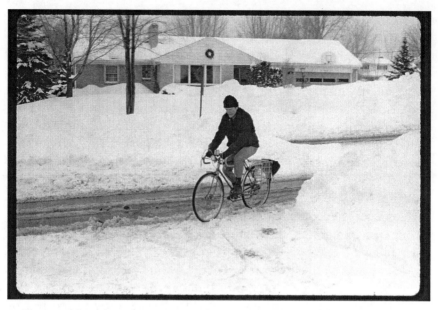

The snowbanks are evident as I return home from work (Winter, 1976)

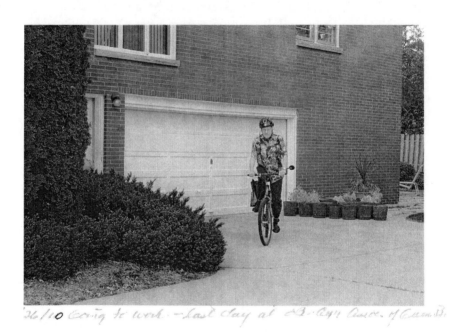

My last day of work in my Green Bay office (May, 2010)

if we could take the $1700 from the insurance company without having the car repaired. The insurance adjuster agreed to that arrangement.

After a few years, Sweetie applied duct tape to the weakened rear-side panels to prevent them from becoming detached. We made the calculation that the $1700 received 15 years ago, invested and compounded (doubling every seven years) was now $6800 and in another seven years would be $13,600, almost enough for a new car.

Sweetie's car has become a conversation piece, especially when we drive to in-state medical meetings. Last July at the meeting of the ACOG's Wisconsin section at the Kalahari Resort in Wisconsin Dells, Dr. Jaeger and his wife Nancy scurried to find their camera to photograph our oddity as we drove by. Having packed the camera away already, they vowed to be ready to open the shutter at the duct-taped car the next time we met.

We have always believed that automobiles were to be used to transport people from point A to point B rather than for all of the reasons for which they are advertised on television. Efficiency and the effect on the environment have been our major considerations when choosing an automobile. The color of our next car will be influenced by what colors are available in duct tape! Our current gray Honda Civic is a perfect match for the silvery duct tape.

My wife continues to purchase a fuel-efficient automobile every fifteen to eighteen years, which when driven 55 mph, provides 45 miles to the gallon for highway driving. Her current 1995 Honda Civic has 152,000 miles registered and has, to date, had no mechanical problems. Our environmental goal is to use each automobile and other possessions until they truly wear out.

The economy and its effect on the environment

As I write this chapter in 2010, the U.S. is suffering from a rather severe recent economic recession that began in 2008. Recessions appear to be inevitable in countries that depend on the free enterprise system. The way democratic countries attempt to prevent or recover from a recession is to stimulate more spending on goods and services. Both of the major political parties in the U.S. appear to be addicted to the concept that we need an annual growth rate of 3-4% in the gross national product (GNP) to prevent or escape from a recession. The GNP measures the total amount of the value of goods and services calculated every three months and annually. We seem to have a monumental contradiction between the annual growth of 3-4% in goods and services and the concepts recommended by Paul Ehrlich and ZPG to decrease wastefulness in our use of natural resources and limit the polluting of our environment.

Incidentally, income for senior citizens (age 65 and above) increased by 5.6% during the first two years since the beginning of the recent recession while the unemployment rate hovered between 9 and 10% and many children remained hungry. This demonstrates the power of the senior citizens' lobby. I do not pretend to be a trained economist, but I do have some questions from the perspective of an ordinary citizen: 1) Can growth go on forever? 2) Does the mind-set that the GNP has to increase accelerate the use of our natural resources? 3) Is an individual's goal to save for future needs unpatriotic? 4) Is there any way for the U.S. economy to be maintained without depending on an annual growth of 3-4%? 5) What percent of the annual GNP increase comes from manufacturing? 6) What percent of the increase comes from services?

The manufacturing of goods accelerates the use of natural resources, increases pollution, and upsets the balance of trade payments. The provision of services has none of the above disadvantages that result from manufacturing growth.

Zero Population Growth (ZPG)

During the end of the 1960s and throughout the 1970s, I and many other fellow citizens became concerned about the dangers of over population. This concern was heightened by Ehrlich's *The Population Bomb* and the formation of Zero Population Growth (ZPG) chapters across the United States. Our own Wisconsin U.S. Senator Gaylord Nelson had helped create our nation's first Earth Day in 1970, planting the seeds of a growing environmental movement that began to recognize the great strain that our increasing population placed on our natural resources.

During the early summer of 1970, I, along with other Green Bay citizens and UWGB faculty members, founded a local chapter of Zero Population Growth (ZPG). I was subsequently elected as the first president. An organizational meeting was held May 15, 1970. The discussions at this meeting were described in a May 16, 1970 *Green Bay Press Gazette* article authored by Sarah Alden Watke with the catchy title, "Group Zeroes in on Population Problem."

By Sarah Alden Watke, *Press-Gazette* staff writer, May 16, 1970

The questions ranged from the cost of adopting a baby to the status of abortion in Wisconsin. But panelists interested in organizing a local chapter of Zero Population Growth (ZPG) kept the tone cool at an informational meeting Friday night.

About 140 persons attended the session at the YMCA. Some 70 indicated they would become members.

Dr. Herbert Sandmire, a Green Bay obstetrician-gynecologist, gave the main talk with John Shier, philosophy professor at the University of Wisconsin, Green Bay, moderating. The Rev. John Decker, a Green Bay minister, and Dr. John Beaton, dean of the university's college of human biology, were the other panelists.

Sandmire said there is no disagreement that ultimate stabilization of population is necessary because within 600 years there would be 1 person per square yard of the earth's surface. This country's population is now doubling every 65 years, the world's every 35 years.

The disagreement, he indicated, is over when stabilization is necessary, when it is desirable and what methods should be used to achieve it.

This country's birth rate is now 17 per thousand annually compared with a death rate of 9 per 1000 annually, Sandmire said. The birth rates require focus "since we're not interested in increasing the death rates."

He drew queries, however, about how his abortion views compared with those of author Paul Ehrlich.

Ehrlich, he answered, "comes from a more sheltered environment than I. Doctors generally do not like abortion as a method of population control. We prefer preventing conceptions to preventing birth – and there is a difference."

He said later that the greatest impact of legalized abortion laws would not be on the population but on the one million women who have them annually.

"Any arguments favoring abortion should be in support of individuals who have good medical care for all other surgical procedures but are forced to go underground for this particular procedure," he said.

"It is often said that men make the laws. I wonder if all men having hernia repairs had the same persons who now do abortions, how long it would be before the laws would change."

This drew applause and some verbal expression of support. He had to add, though, that until the Supreme Court rules on constitu-

75

tionality of laws, anyone performing an abortion during the inter-vening period could be prosecuted. And a Washington, D.C. case will reach the Supreme Court before a Wisconsin case, he said.

As nationwide interest in preventing future problems resulting from overpopulation grew in the 1970s, so did my own passion for this cause. My efforts were recognized by the Wisconsin ZPG with its Humanitarian Award, which I received in May of 1974:

> *For release Wednesday, May 1, 1974, 3 PM*
> *Dr. Herbert Sandmire, winner of ZPG Humanitarian Award*
> *Madison - - A Green Bay physician, Dr. Herbert F. Sandmire, was among six persons honored by the Wisconsin Confederation of Zero Population Growth (ZPG) today at an annual awards confer-ence held at the Wisconsin Center on the University of Wisconsin campus in Madison.*
>
> *Dr. Sandmire received the group's major citation, the Humani-tarian Award, for "his many years of active involvement in obtaining better health care for women."*
>
> *Activist Awards went to three Wisconsin women, Rev. Eleanor Yeo, Milwaukee, for her work with the Clergy Consultation Service on Problem Pregnancies; Beatrice Kabler, Madison, who is president of Wisconsin Citizens for Family Planning; and Joan Allan of the Madison chapter of the National Organization for Women for her volunteer lobbying on behalf of women's rights.*
>
> *A couple, Jeff and Jill Dean, Madison, received the Family of the Year Award.*
>
> *ZPG's citation for Dr. Sandmire continued, in part: "We honor Dr. Sandmire for a great variety of services to individuals, to his com-munity, and to the state. We note especially his initial help in fund-ing Green Bay Planned Parenthood and his service as a founding member of its board of advisors and of its volunteer medical staff."*
>
> *Other activities of Dr. Sandmire's cited by ZPG are:*
> * *his volunteer work in lecturing at Bellin Memorial Hospi-tal School of Nursing*
> * *his regular guest lectures, without salary, at the University of Wisconsin, Green Bay*
> * *his service as a University of Wisconsin Medical School pre-ceptor, another volunteer teaching activity in which senior medical students spend 8 weeks of their last year of medical school with him.*

- *His acceptance of all referrals of Green Bay Free Clinic patients for gynecological and obstetrical care*
- *His professional studies and publications including one relating to oral contraceptives which received worldwide attention in the press and has been disseminated in family planning programs overseas by the U. S. Agency for International Development*
- *an article relating to avoidable maternal deaths in Wisconsin which focused professional attention on that critical problem and received wide notice*
- *his 50 speeches and appearances on behalf of ZPG and population problems*
- *his appearances at legislative hearings and his work within medical societies for the availability of birth control, sterilization and abortion.*

Dr. Sandmire's professional memberships include the Wisconsin Society of Obstetrics and Gynecology, of which he is an immediate past president; the Wisconsin State Medical Society and its Maternal Mortality Study Committee; the American Medical Association; the American College of Surgeons; the American College of Obstetricians and Gynecologists; the Central Association of Obstetricians and Gynecologists; the Iowa Society of Obstetricians and Gynecologists (honorary); the Brown County Medical Association.

ZPG also noted a contribution of Dr. Sandmire's outside its scope of honor, but of general interest: He has been a financial backer and a manager and coach of a Little League baseball team for seven years. As manager of the Allouez Orioles, he saw his team become Champions of the League in 1972 and 1973.

The ZPG award prompted Dr. Keettel, Chairman of the University of Iowa Department of Ob/Gyn, to once again try to recruit me to his department.

The University of Iowa
Department of Obstetrics and Gynecology
Iowa City, Iowa 52242

Dear Herb,

It was pleasant chatting with you at Dr. Bradbury's retirement activities. I am sorry that I did not have the opportunity to visit more with you. I have read with great interest about your recent honor. It certainly is well deserved and commend you on all the community pro-jects that you have been involved in. This is a great tribute to you and I only wish that our former residents were this public spirited and community oriented. My only regret is that you have not seen fit to use your talents in academic medicine where I think your impact would be even greater than it is in the private sector.

Again, my heartfelt congratulations to a job well done. With kindest personal regards.

Sincerely, Wm. Keettel, Chrm.

I was flattered by his comments, but still believed that I could make a bigger impact in private practice.

CHAPTER 13

Planned Parenthood / more publications / family planning comes of age

IN FEBRUARY OF 1971, Planned Parenthood opened a birth control counseling office in Green Bay, and I was a member of its founding Board of Directors. The office provided examinations as well as birth control services. I served as the physician on duty one evening a week for a few years. Following my years of service, the Green Bay office became staffed with nurse practitioners and physician assistants. In October of 2008, I began to work at the Appleton Planned Parenthood Clinic, and I continue to this date one or two days a week.

These were exciting times for a young doctor developing a successful medical clinic while keeping his finger on the pulse of the academic world. I was thrilled to receive a Citation of Special Merit in 1969 from the State Medical Society of Wisconsin for my presentation on the intrauterine contraceptive device (IUD) at the Society's annual meeting in Milwaukee, Wisconsin.

The following year, I presented our clinical practice's "Experience with 15,000 consecutive pap smears" at the American College of Obstetricians and Gynecologists' District VI meeting 1970 in St. Paul, Minnesota. The paper was ultimately published in April of 1972 in the *Wisconsin Medical Journal*.

The worldwide attention devoted to what we thought to be a relatively unimportant paper was truly beyond all expectations and belief. Crystal and I drove home from the meeting in St. Paul the afternoon of November 14, 1970 – the meeting having ended at noon that day. We were on a tight schedule as we were to play bridge at the home of Jim and Helen Wright that evening. We quickly changed clothes and were off to the Wrights, about three blocks away. At their home, we received the first of many newspaper reporter calls from across the United States, forwarded to us by our baby sitter. The reporters calling were seeking further information on my presentation in St. Paul, in particular the finding that the use of oral contraceptives did not increase the risk for cancer of the uterine cervix, contrary to the findings of a previously published New York study. The Associated Press picked up the report of the *Minneapolis Star* reporter, and later I was told that more than 400 newspapers in the United States and Canada published the article describing my presentation. Friends and family sent copies from their newspapers from Detroit, Denver, the Canadian *Hamilton Spectator* and numerous others. The United States Agency for International Development sent a description of my paper to all of its worldwide offices and family planning centers.

What caused all of the excitement?

The article in the *Minneapolis Star* on November 14, 1970 follows:_

Study shows cancer not enhanced by "pill," by Gordon Slovat, (*Minneapolis Star* Staff Writer)

The use of oral contraceptive pills does not increase a woman's chance of getting cancer of the cervix, according to a Green Bay obstetrician-gynecologist, Dr. Herbert F. Sandmire, one of three specialists in the care of women at the multi-specialty Beaumont Clinic in Green Bay, presented the findings at an upper Midwest conference of the American College of Obstetricians and Gynecologists in the St. Paul Hilton Hotel. His findings were based on the results of 15,000 Pap smears – a simple test for symptoms of cancer of the cervix, the lower part of the uterus – on Beaumont Clinic patients from 1960 to 1969. Dr. Sandmire said the patients were generally a "homogeneous group" – mostly white, middle class with similar social outlook and mores.

The finding contradicts a New York study which indicated that cancer of the uterus rate was higher among pill users than among those not on the pill, Dr. Sandmire said. But he added that he believes the New York study was faulty.

In the Pap smear a physician removes some secretions from the upper part of the vagina and from the surface of the cervix and sends them to a lab for examination. Cancer of the cervix is one of the most common types of cancer in women.

Dr. Sandmire reported that 28 cancer cases were found from among 12,000 Pap smears from women not on oral contraceptives or a rate of one per 428 Pap smears.

Six cancers were found among pill-taking women from whom 3,000 Pap smears were taken, or an almost identical rate of one per 500 Pap smears, he said.

He said the New York study probably was invalid because of the type of women who selected the pill at the family planning center used for the investigation.

The women were of a type who probably had sexual intercourse early in life with a variety of partners, a style of living which some doctors believe increases a woman's chance of getting cervical cancer, he said.

Women with a middle-class outlook are more apt to start their birth control efforts with a diaphragm because they are not likely to have as many partners, he said.

He said he suspects that the diaphragm may offer protection against contamination which may be cancer-encouraging.

Oral contraceptives had only been available for ten years at the time of our report. With their use still considered controversial, and their alleged potential to cause cervical cancer, our study attracted wide interest from the media. And while some had moral misgivings about the use of the contraceptive pill, I saw it as one solution to the population explosion resulting from the post-World War II baby boom.

Family planning comes of age

Helping to establish the safety of birth control pills was another thing I felt I could do to address the bigger problem of over population. Furthermore, I saw this easy-to-use method of birth control as a way to avoid maternal mortality as well. My work in this area culminated in my eighth published paper, entitled "Family planning comes of age," which also appeared in the *Wisconsin Medical Journal* in April of 1972. The data from this study was accumulated from the findings of the Wisconsin Maternal Mortality Study Committee.

The article was written because of my observation of the frequent deaths occurring in women inappropriately pregnant. In fact, thirty two of the last forty eight consecutive deaths reviewed by the study committee occurred in women who had serious and important reasons for avoiding pregnancy. These reasons consisted of serious medical problems which could be life – threatening during a pregnancy: seven women already had four or more children along with serious medical problems, six women already had four or more children, twelve women left 70 children motherless (surveys at the time before publication of this article indicated that only 20 percent of women with four children desire another pregnancy), and seven women had unwanted pregnancies, five of whom died from complications of an illegal abortion performed by non-physicians.

Pregnancies occurred in some of these women because of failure of or failure to use contraceptives – women who should have been offered a therapeutic abortion on the basis of their serious underlying medical condition. Tragically, one of the deaths occurred in a woman whose request for a therapeutic abortion was denied even though she already had five children and severe hypertension of several years duration. She was later admitted to the hospital in a comatose condition due to a massive brain hemorrhage. One day prior to her death, she delivered a still-born infant. I believed at the time (1972), and still do, that the greatest potential for further reduction of maternal deaths rests with the prevention of inappropriate pregnancies.

CHAPTER 14

January 22, 1973

WHILE THE GROWING use of "the pill" stirred debate on the religious and political landscape, any controversy associated with it was soon dwarfed by what came next. On January 22, 1973, the United States Supreme Court issued a ruling in *Roe v. Wade* that a woman could not be prevented from exercising her constitutional right to have her pregnancy terminated. Therefore, abortions could be performed in every state without fear of prosecution, since all laws prohibiting abortion were ruled unconstitutional. This presented a dilemma for obstetricians and gynecologists: would they or would they not provide legally allowed abortions?

At the Beaumont Clinic, the majority of the partners believed that abortion services should not be provided by its obstetricians and gynecologists. This required Dr. Austin and me to abandon our patients, some of whom were long-standing, if we withheld or were unwilling to perform the requested abortion. Dr. Austin and I "voted with our feet," deciding to leave a Clinic that failed to recognize a woman's constitutional right to have her pregnancy terminated. We were faced with a degree of uncertainty as to whether our decision for women's rights would negatively impact our economic well-being. I remember the wife of a surgeon living on our street predicting that our children would probably go to bed hungry as a result of their father's decision. However, such dire predictions did not deter us from what we felt was the right decision, regardless of any loss of income that might occur. As it turned out, our ability to attract patients never decreased, and our income, after moving from the Beaumont Clinic, increased significantly.

Jane Doe sues Bellin

The historic landmark decision by the U.S. Supreme Court was hailed by physicians who provide healthcare for women, most of the public and also those who treasure individual freedoms. During April of 1973, I assisted a patient in her suit against Bellin Hospital for violating her constitutional right to have her pregnancy terminated. Since Bellin hospital is affiliated with the Wisconsin Conference of the United Methodist Church, I presumed they (the hospital) would have policies similar to the church on the performance of abortion. To my surprise, the Bellin Board of Trustees, exclusively comprised of older, well-to-do men, ultimately prevented my patient from receiving an abortion at the hospital.

Excerpts from the *Green Bay Press Gazette* article of April 27, 1973 describe the reasons for the lawsuit:

Bellin Sued for Blocking Abortion

Dr. Herbert Sandmire Thursday sued Bellin Memorial Hospital in federal court at Milwaukee charging that the Green Bay hospital refused to allow an abortion to be performed in its facilities in violation of a patient's rights.

The suit said the refusal violated the constitutional rights of a patient identified only as Jane Doe of Shawano. Sandmire's attorney, Paul Jonjak of Sturgeon Bay, said the suit asks for both a preliminary injunction to prevent the hospital from interfering with this case and a permanent injunction to prevent the hospital from interfering with the Green Bay doctor's practice.

The injunction requests are based on a U.S. Supreme Court decision in January which said that abortion in the first trimester is a matter "between doctor and patient only," according to Jonjak....

Dr. Sandmire's patient had an abortion appointment at a Madison clinic, Midwest Medical Center, for April 9, but a snowstorm that day prevented her from keeping it, the suit says. Sandmire then determined that her pregnancy, which dated from about Feb. 4, was too far advanced for clinic surgery and required hospital facilities, the complaint says.... The suit says he examined her April 19 and decided the abortion should be performed before May 4 when the first trimester of pregnancy ends....

The information was made public before Bellin was served with the papers, according to both Bellin Hospital administrator, Dan Smith and Sandmire's attorney. Jonjak said he filed the papers at 3 p.m. Thursday and is now waiting for a case date and to learn whether Judge John Reynolds or Judge Myron Gordon will try the case in U.S. District Court. Bellin will be served the papers as soon as he knows the date, Jonjak explained....

Smith, Bellin Administrator, declined to comment when asked why Bellin, a Methodist hospital, has an abortion policy that is more conservative than that adopted by the general conference of the United Methodist Church. Methodists have also testified in favor of liberalized abortion reforms at various public hearings, including congressional committees.

The American Civil Liberties Union (ACLU), an organization known for advocating and protecting individual rights, was invited to assist in the suit against Bellin Hospital. Their financial and moral support, as well as their dissemination of accurate information to the public, was deeply appreciated. The ACLU's role and views were reported in a Tuesday, May 1, 1973 *Green Bay Press Gazette* article, excerpts of which follow:

ACLU Says Abortion Suit Seeks To Give Law to All

The American Civil Liberties Union says it joined an abortion suit against Bellin Memorial Hospital in an effort to make certain the law of the land is carried out.

The Northeastern Wisconsin Chapter of the ACLU is a party to a suit filed by Dr. Herbert Sandmire who says he was denied permission to perform an abortion at Bellin hospital on a woman in the first trimester of pregnancy. A hearing will be held at 10 a.m. Wednesday before Judge Myron Gordon in the U.S. District Court in Milwaukee.

"Now that the United States Supreme Court has settled the issue of legality of abortions, it is important that all individuals and institutions in the country work to make sure that the law of the land is carried out," said David Galaty, chairman of the Northeastern Wisconsin chapter, ACLU.

The Supreme Court has stated that a woman in the first trimester of pregnancy and her physician are legally entitled to medically terminate that pregnancy. "There is no question about this," according to Galaty.

In Green Bay, however, no hospital permits use of its facilities for termination of pregnancy. Green Bay hospitals have received large sums of money from the federal government to build their facilities. "They are public institutions designed to serve the medical needs of all persons in this area, despite the fact that they are administered by private organizations," Galaty's statement said.

"There is no basis for a hospital, which is supported by public money, to refuse to perform legal medical services for which it is equipped. It is as if hospitals in this area refused to allow appendectomies to be performed on their premises, thereby causing great, potential harm to those with appendicitis."

"The state Medical Society," Galaty noted, "has affirmed every year since 1970 its position that a physician should have a clear right 'to abort the unquickened product of conception within the dictates of his own training, experience and conscience.'"

In the final analysis, the Bellin hospital policies allowed it to discriminate against patients with certain needs rather than allowing discrimination based on religious beliefs, skin color or sexual orientation. The proper interpretation, which should be evident to all, is that Bellin sought to justify its policies which discriminate against a class of patients based on those patients' needs. Sadly, as the reader will see at the very end of this story, discrimination against classes of patients is alive and well in the United States, despite the 1973 *Roe v. Wade* Supreme Court ruling, the battles for social justice in the 1960s, and the passage of civil rights legislation.

District Judge Gordon ruled that Bellin must allow abortions in its facility, but Bellin representatives were 100 percent mobilized to accomplish their mission of protecting their discriminatory policies and preventing this young, unsophisticated woman from exercising her legal right to terminate her pregnancy. They "proudly" petitioned the 7th U.S. Circuit Court of Appeals in Chicago to review Judge Myron Gordon's ruling.

If the hospital had not challenged Judge Gordon's ruling, the hospital's discrimination policy would no longer have prevailed and the interest in the issues involved would have diminished over time (everyone wins). But the hospital representatives were on a mission. The hospital's petition of Judge Gordon's ruling and request for a review by the Appeals Court can best be described by the following excerpts from the May 4th, 1973, *Green Bay Press Gazette* article:

Bellin Granted Stay on Abortion Order, *by Sarah Watke, Press Gazette Staff Writer*

Drama mounted Wednesday in a Green Bay lawsuit – the first of its kind in Wisconsin – when a Chicago federal appeals court halted an earlier federal court order directing Bellin Memorial Hospital to allow an abortion to be performed in its facilities. Judge John Paul Stevens of the 7th U.S. Circuit Court of Appeals in Chicago granted a stay of a preliminary injunction handed down a few hours earlier by Judge Myron Gordon of U.S. District Court in Milwaukee, pending a hearing expected today.

At issue is the question of whether a court may order a hospital to allow an abortion to be performed, whether the hospital is a private institution which may do as it wishes or a public institution and an agent of the state. The suit, filed by Dr. Herbert Sandmire on behalf of a patient identified only as Jane Doe of Shawano, contends the alleged interference of the hospital is a state action because of government funding of hospitals and governmental controls.

The lawsuit against Bellin is believed to be the first in the nation dealing with the issue of a hospital's authority to set abortion policy, even though the U.S. Supreme Court has already settled one question, ruling that a woman has a legal right to an abortion in her first trimester of pregnancy. Neither federal court serving Wisconsin has ever had a case challenging a hospital's abortion policy, according to the two clerks of the U.S. District Courts serving the eastern and western parts of the state. Sources such as the American Civil Liberties Union also report no knowledge of such cases in their headquarters in cities like New York and Chicago. There has been at least one case involving a sterilization request in which a hospital in Montana was ordered to allow its facilities to be used, sources said.

Dr. Sandmire's suit asks [for] a preliminary injunction on behalf of his patient because he says that she must have the abortion by Friday, May 4, to come within her first trimester. The woman requires hospital facilities, he contends, because it is too late in her trimester for her to have the operation in a clinic. An original April 9th abortion appointment at a Madison clinic had to be cancelled due to a snowstorm.

Smith, the hospital administrator, said the hospital won the stay of the preliminary injunction by leaving their prepared materials with the Chicago appeals court and learned of the status upon returning to Green Bay Wednesday night.

The next step in our quest seeking justice and fair treatment for Jane Doe involved a petition to the U.S. Supreme Court. This was described in a Saturday, May 5th, 1973 *Green Bay Press Gazette* article:

Supreme Court Decides in Bellin's Favor

The U.S. Supreme Court has decided Bellin Memorial Hospital doesn't have to allow use of its facilities for an abortion – at least until further court arguments are heard. The highest court in the land Friday issued an order granting Bellin's request for a further hearing in a Chicago appeals court to settle the abortion suit.

The high court denied the motion of Dr. Herbert Sandmire on behalf of an unidentified Shawano woman to vacate a Thursday order of the 7th U.S. Circuit Court of Appeals in Chicago....

Supreme Court Justice William H. Rehnquist, who has jurisdiction over the 7th circuit court, declined to handle the matter himself, which was his prerogative and took it before the full court Friday. The vote was 7-0 to deny the motion, with Justices Byron White and Thurgood Marshall taking no part, according to James Blondell, assistant clerk of the Supreme Court.

The high court didn't give a written opinion with its two-sentence order, and did not explain whether Justices White and Marshall were present during proceedings....

Sandmire had won Supreme Court consideration of the preliminary orders on one-day notice by claiming that the woman needed to have the abortion by today and that medical risk to her would be greater in a later abortion due to a need to change to a different, saline abortion method. The risk, although still small, is 10 times higher, according to an affidavit filed in the case by Dr. Sandmire....

Friday, the trimester argument and the plaintiff's success in obtaining Supreme Court involvement on short notice commanded all the attention. But the case still involves other crucial legal issues, according to attorneys and principals.

Is the hospital a private institution or a state agent, because of receiving government funds and regulations? Is the hospital interfering with the patient's right to medical services that are available, or is the hospital a private institution which may do as it wishes?

The Bellin case is the first in Wisconsin and believed to be the first in the nation which seeks to compel a hospital to allow its facilities for an abortion.

In the end, we failed to overturn Bellin's discriminatory abortion policy. In essence, it was a classic case of the powerful triumphing over the powerless. In addition, the mission to protect Bellin's policy was controlled by middle-aged or older men who would never request or be in need of an abortion. The intensity and boldness with which these older men pursued their mission to prevent this woman from having a safe abortion at Bellin astonished, baffled and disappointed me: organizing a team of lawyers, flying legal papers to Washington, making themselves available for travel to Washington within four hours, and appealing Judge Gordon's decision. Comparatively speaking, they pursued their mission with the same zeal or intensity I would imagine for a team of CIA agents chasing down a suspected terrorist. I still wonder today whether Bellin officials are proud of their actions and what they accomplished? It seems senseless to use healthcare dollars that come from patients to perpetuate discriminatory policies – not to mention the fact that when all was said and done, Jane Doe was forced to have the more dangerous, second-trimester abortion in Madison.

CHAPTER 15

Birth Control, Conferences, and the Easy Riders

IN 1975, MY partners, Drs. Stephen Austin and Richard Bechtel, and I published a follow-up study to our 1972 paper entitled "Experience with 15,000 pap smears." This earlier paper received extensive media coverage because it provided reassuring information that the birth control pill did not increase the woman's risk for cervical cancer. Given the extensive use of the contraceptive pill around the world, we thought that it was important to confirm our earlier findings with a study involving a larger number of women taking the pill over a longer period of time.

We presented this follow-up study at the 1975 annual meeting of CAOG and published it as "Carcinoma of the cervix in oral contraceptive steroid and IUD users and nonusers" in the June 1976 issue of the *American Journal of Obstetrics and Gynecology*. We again found no increase in risk of cervical cancer in users of birth control pills. Similarly, we found no increase in cervical cancer risk for intrauterine contraceptive device (IUD) users either. As our article's abstract explained, "A trial of 40,211 cytologic examinations and subsequent diagnostic procedures resulted in the diagnosis of carcinoma of the cervix in 76 patients. The 76 patients did not demonstrate any variations in use of oral contraceptive steroids or intrauterine devices when compared to 780 randomly selected control patients."

One month later, Austin, Bechtel, and I published a related paper entitled "Experience with 40,000 pap smears" in the July 1976 issue of *Obstetrics and Gynecology*. The most significant finding of this study was that 25 of the 76 carcinomas were diagnosed in patients with only atypical (class II) smears, indicating that all patients with persistent atypical smears also require evaluation by tissue examination.

I presented my next paper, "Minilaparotomy tubal sterilization," at the annual CAOG meeting in October of 1977 at Biloxi, Mississippi. This study was subsequently published in the June 1978 issue of the *American Journal of Obstetrics and Gynecology*. Its major conclusion was that "the minilaparotomy procedure provides the safest and best current method of tubal sterilization for the patient who is not massively obese. This finding had important implications for practicing gynecologists, and as such, I presented it again at the Sixth Annual Meeting of Ambulatory Surgical Care in Salt Lake City in February of 1980, at the annual meeting of the Wisconsin Society of Obstetricians and Gynecologists in Baraboo, Wisconsin in July of 1980, and at the annual meeting of ACOG District VI in Rapid City, South Dakota in August of 1983.

The journal *Family Practice Recertification* subsequently invited me to write an article with a similar title that appeared in their January 1982 issue. The thanks I received for the manuscript also included a check for $300 – the first and only time I ever received payment for an article.

By this time we had become reacquainted with motorcycles as a part of our lives. Any memories I had of crashing my older brother Ty's motorcycle and ripping open my knee at age 14, were too remote to keep the Peter Fonda in me from getting back on the saddle. Crystal checked the Post Office schedule to determine how long it would take two suitcases to travel by regular mail from Green Bay to Rapid City, South Dakota – five days, we learned. We sent them so that they would arrive there one day before we zoomed in on our motorcycle. They were waiting for us behind the counter as we checked into the hotel.

We enjoyed exploring the Badlands, the Black Hills, and Monument National Park before the meeting began. The temperature in the Badlands was 104 degrees, which was tolerable until the moment we stopped and had no breeze in our faces to cool off.

On Saturday at noon, the meeting ended and we began the trip home, intending to ride a few hours before finding a motel. We drove and we drove until I began to think we were going to sleep on the ground, but finally we found a motel with one room available.

About that same time we went on another long motorcycle trip to visit my sister Corinne in North Carolina. We would often ride for one or two hours before breakfast to avoid having to ride for several hours in a row later in the day. Once, when we stopped at a fancy hotel for

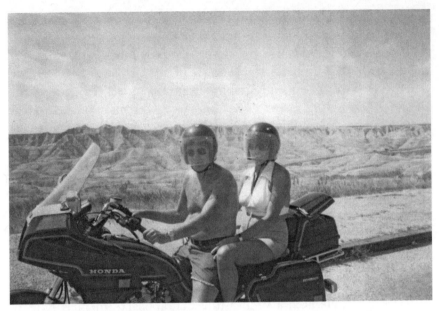

Enjoying the Badlands enroute to the 1983 meeting of
ACOG District VI in Rapid City, South Dakota

breakfast, Crystal went in while I bought a *Wall Street Journal* from the dispenser. When I came in to the restaurant, I asked the hostess in a booming voice, "Have any of our gang arrived?" Quick as a whistle, she retorted, "You can't fool me Mister, your wife said you were out there getting a *Wall Street Journal!*"

The exhilaration of travel by motorcycle prompted us to take more long-distance trips in the 1980s, two of which were to Helena, Montana, where our daughters Cheryl and Yvonne lived at that time, and one that was a ten-day trip home from Cheryl's wedding in Santa Barbara, California. Cheryl had purchased a medium-sized motorcycle for that purpose. We visited friends and relatives for four of the nine overnight stays. The first eight days were pleasant and uneventful, but on the ninth day we awakened to a rainy, cold morning. We started out from Kansas City, where we had stayed overnight with our son Kevin and his wife Karen, and headed toward Des Moines, Iowa. We soon discovered that our gortex rain gear was not waterproof as advertised in the 50-degree weather. The combination of being soaked, the low temperature, and the effect of the wind attacking our bodies made us more than cold. We stopped along the way at fast food restaurants to warm up, using the bathroom hand dryers for heat.

Crystal suggested we rent a car and a U-Haul trailer for the motorcycle. I objected to that plan, and the rain had stopped as we approached Des Moines. Before she could start divorce talk, I promised her we would stop at a Sears store in Des Moines and buy her dry clothes. We did, and the rest of the trip was much better.

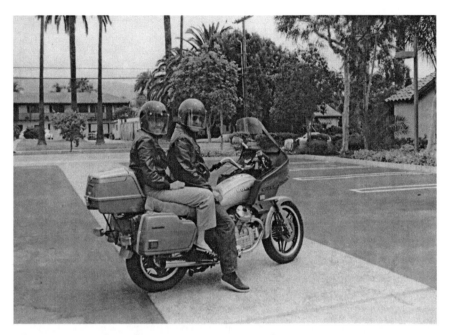

Starting home from Santa Barbara following Cheryl's wedding. We stayed with friends and relatives for four of the nine nights. (May 27, 1985)

CHAPTER 16

Two awards to the Sandmires

ON MAY 1, 1974 Wisconsin Zero Population Growth (ZPG) organization issued a news release indicating that I was the recipient of their Humanitarian Award. Five days later, our daughter Yvonne received Sportswoman of the Year award at the 13th annual Elks Sports Award dinner in Green Bay. Elks Club officials noted that "Over the past two years, Yvonne Sandmire is undefeated in state gymnastics competition. Her coach at the Green Bay YMCA, Cameron McCain, claims she is the premier girls' gymnast in the state of Wisconsin and the best ever produced in the city." With glowing praise, McCain says, 'She is the type of kid any coach would love to have on his team.' An 18-year old senior at Preble High School, Yvonne competes in the balance beam, uneven parallel bars, vaulting and floor exercise. And next year she expects to continue in competitive gymnastics at Arizona State University, where she has received an athletic scholarship.

Hearing of these awards, former Wisconsin Badger football player Roger Dornburg and his wife wrote a particularly nice letter to us, saying that they "want[ed] to congratulate you on the recent honors received by Yvonne and Dr. Sandmire. I have admired not only Yvonne's ability and talent but that radiant look of peace and contentment. For a long time I have prayed that our girls develop so beautifully. We realize it has been the result of a family environment and effort. The respect and gratitude that our family holds for Dr. Sandmire and his talent and ability makes us very happy that he received public recognition for the very thing we have known for many years. We thank all of you for giving our community these two dedicated individuals."

As is a father's right to brag about his kids, I was pleased when *Green Bay Press Gazette* sports reporter Don Langenkamp also captured Yvonne's exuberant personality in his article of January 26, 1978, writing that:

> *One of the toughest hypothetical assignments I can conjure up in my mind would be to find someone who would say anything bad about Yvonne Sandmire. In fact, it's more than tough. It's virtually impossible.*
>
> *Sandmire gets nothing but superlatives from Cameron McCain, her gymnastics coach during her YMCA days, to Don Robinson, who heads up the program at Arizona State.*
>
> *After interviewing her, it's easy to see why. She has a radiant personality along with boundless energy and confidence.*
>
> *And all those qualities are funneled into one thing: gymnastics.*
>
> *"She's absolutely super," says Robinson. "She's the one who gets kids excited about gymnastics. She's a big reason for much of the program's success here. She helps in teaching gymnastics and when we want to promote our program, we can always depend on her to help."*
>
> *"She was the groundbreaker here," says Mc Cain. "She was a real pioneer for gymnastics in Green Bay."*
>
> *When Sandmire was a member of the YMCA team, she was the name in area – even state – gymnastics. But when she arrived at Arizona State, she was just another talented gal proficient on things like a balance beam, uneven bars and the like.*
>
> *But ASU quickly found she was more than that. She has an almost evangelistic feeling about her sport. She has just embarked on her last year of competition at ASU and the fervor hasn't diminished.*
>
> *While Sandmire plays down her ability, she has made all-conference the past two years. Arizona State has won the conference title every year since she's been there. At the national tournament last year, ASU finished seventh and Sandmire had the second highest score on her team.*
>
> *Gymnastics and Sandmire aren't about to part company. She is aiming for a job with a gymnastics equipment manufacturer and she'd like to coach on the side. While she has devoted a good share of her young life to a demanding sport, she feels far from being deprived. "I wouldn't change anything if I had to do it over again. I got to travel to a lot of places and meet a lot of nice people."*

CHAPTER 17

The first test tube baby

TUESDAY, JULY 25, 1978 was a historic day in medicine. On that day, Louise Brown, the world's first "test tube baby" was born. British biologist Robert Edwards and the late gynecologist Patrick Steptoe had removed an unfertilized egg from the mother's ovary and fertilized it with her husband's sperm in a laboratory test tube. They then successfully implanted the fertile egg in her uterus. Just recently, Robert Edwards received the 2010 Nobel Prize in medicine for his amazing feat. Nonetheless, at the time, the public response to this breakthrough was mixed. *Green Bay Press Gazette* reporter Sarah Watke, looking for local reaction to this medical milestone, interviewed Catholic priest Roy Klister and me for an article in her paper, some of which went like this:

> *The birth of a baby that was conceived in a test tube "isn't complicated morally or medically" in the eyes of a local Protestant gynecologist, Dr. Herbert Sandmire.*
>
> *But Msgr. Roy Klister, vice chancellor of the Catholic Diocese of Green Bay, sees the event and its implications as "terribly complex."*
>
> *Both see the successful birth as less controversial than artificial insemination, however, because the egg and the sperm came from a married couple.*
>
> *Klister agreed with Sandmire and the Rev. Kenneth Keller, associate pastor at First United Methodist, that the marriage of the parents involved "puts it into a different moral perspective." But the priest had other objections.*
>
> *Sandmire said "It is simply a method for getting around a patient's disability, the blockage of her Fallopian tubes. It is using her*

egg and her husband's sperm to produce a conception. Since society holds it appropriate for a wife and husband's egg and sperm to unite, it was accomplished with the assistance needed."

The physician said he doesn't see any great danger of deformed babies. "However, if it should occur it wouldn't be a precedent. There are harmful effects (within the uterus) from radiation and sometimes drugs. Only through careful analysis of data can the danger be determined," he said.

Sandmire added that the patients have the right to take the risk, however, and make an informed request for the procedure when it becomes available.

He said that of 5 percent of women who are infertile for various reasons, about one half to one percent have blocked Fallopian tubes like Mrs. Brown.

Klister disagreed with Sandmire's conclusions. He said "it is fortuitous that the delivery did result in a healthy normal baby. Right now this is highly experimental with human life, you are in danger of taking the control out of its natural context of family, etc."

CHAPTER 18

$\mathcal{U}.\mathcal{S}.$ $\mathcal{H}$ealth care costs

IN ADDITION TO the abortion issue, the escalating costs of health care in the 1970s was a growing concern of mine. I presented my next paper, "Curettage as an office procedure," at the 41st Annual Meeting of the Central Association of Obstetricians and Gynecologists in Scottsdale, Arizona in October of 1973. Subsequently published in the May 1974 issue of the *American Journal of Obstetrics and Gynecology*, this article reported on the health care cost savings available with the performance of curettage (removing the lining of the uterus) in the office rather than the hospital. The accumulated savings for the 561 study patients totaled $182,000. The annual savings nationally, if only half of all curettage procedures were performed in the office, was astronomical: 637,500 cases times an average savings of $325 per case for a total of $211,187,500.

Our growing experience performing this procedure in an outpatient setting led to my next paper, "Curettage in the office," which was published in *Consultant* in August of 1974. The main focus of this article was to describe the techniques for performance of this procedure, the selection of patients, and the recommended safety measures.

The Green Bay Area Free Clinic

In the early to mid-1970s, a free clinic founded by Green Bay internist John Randall opened in Green Bay. The goal of the clinic was to "provide health care services to all populations in need but unable to afford it." The care was delivered by other Green Bay physicians and me. The Green Bay Area Free Clinic acknowledged my work with their "1978 Green Bay Area Free Clinic Physician Award," noting that the Clinic "gratefully recognizes the dedicated personal service given by H. Sandmire MD in furtherance of the clinic's goal of providing health care services to all populations in need and yet unable to afford it. Presented with the gratitude and warm regards of the Board of Directors, the Staff and volunteers and the patients of the Green Bay Area Free Clinic."

I later received the 1979 "Presidential citation of the State Medical Society of Wisconsin" in recognition of my "commitment and devoted service as a volunteer physician to the Green Bay Area Free Clinic for providing medical care to persons in need, thus personifying the high ideals of the medical profession in public service."

The expanded role of the medical assistant in our Ob/Gyn practice

It occurred to me in the early 1970s that there were other ways to reduce the high costs of health care. At this time, a physician shortage was looming across the U.S. medical landscape. It had been known that the Armed Forces had expanded the role of Medical Corpsman, especially on the battlefield. Using that experience as a guide, we initiated a program to train medical assistants for new careers as physician assistants (PAs). The concept was that a PA working under the direct supervision of the physician could perform many of the physician's tasks without sacrificing the quality of care.

In 1971 we started our in-clinic training program, for three physician assistants, which was to run for two years in a progressive fashion. Initially we repeated the entire physical exam performed by our "students," depending on them primarily for assistance in recording the medical history for each patient encounter. At the same time we trained them in the performance of the physical examination, recording their work in a "training book." The supervising physician would grade the examination as either satisfactory or not, specifying in the latter case which components of the examination were not satisfactory. This method allowed us to describe the training process for any licensing agency or other physicians who may be interested in training their PAs.

We found that the trainees often performed some components of the exam better than others. For example, a trainee might require a greater number of checked examinations of the heart or breasts compared to the abdomen or pelvis. Each component was rechecked by the physician until the trainee demonstrated competency in that part of the examination. Thereafter, our PAs were scheduled to perform annual physical examinations.

The history-taking aspect for our "students" was basically unchanged from what they had been doing in our office for the previous four to six years. Our next challenge was to determine which illnesses could be managed independently by the PA. Examples of conditions managed by the PAs included uncomplicated bladder infections, vaginal discharge complaints, menstrual abnormalities for patients under 40 years of age, contraceptive management, and prenatal care for uncomplicated pregnancies.

In 1975 the Wisconsin Department of Regulation and Licensing set up a certifying process and examinations that were available for our clinic-trained PAs. Happily, all three of our trainees passed the certifying examination and continued to work in our office as PAs for the next 30 years, until their retirement at which time they were replaced by formally trained PAs or nurse practitioners. Recognizing the problem (physician shortage) and developing a solution benefitted our patients, the physicians in our office, and the PAs, who with certification commanded higher pay. The use of PAs enabled the physician to see more patients with increased efficiency, thereby reducing healthcare costs.

Somehow Dr. Keettel, chairman of the OB/Gyn department at the University of Iowa became aware of our PA training program and invited me to describe it at their annual postgraduate conference on November 28, 1973:

The University of Iowa
Department of Obstetrics and Gynecology
Iowa City, Iowa 52240

Dear Herb,
It was pleasant talking on the phone and I want to officially invite you as a guest speaker for our postgraduate course to be held on November 28 and 29, 1973.

I would like to have you discuss the matter of nurse assistant and how this has increased the efficiency of the two doctors and really has substituted for the obstetrician and gynecologist who left. You can let me know the title of your presentation as soon as convenient.

I will be anxious to talk more with you in April when you are in Iowa City. With kindest personal regards to you and your wife.

Sincerely, W.C. Keettel MD, Chrm.

I was gratified to experience this reversal of roles, a case of a private practitioner enlightening physicians at a University academic center, rather than the reverse. I later gave the same lecture in Omaha, Nebraska at the ACOG District VI meeting and at the meeting of the Wisconsin Society of Obstetrics and Gynecology at Cable, Wisconsin, in July 1977.

Forgiving an old physician for a temporary lapse of modesty, I will state that training our own PAs at a time when formal PA training programs were non-existent and employing them for 30 years is probably the most significant of my accomplishments, with the possible exception of the development of the Green Bay Surgical Center which opened in January of 1978.

Green Bay Surgical Center

As a further quest to provide low-cost, high-quality health care services, I began planning an ambulatory surgical center in the summer of 1976. When we opened it in January of 1978, our facility was the first free-standing ambulatory surgical center in the state of Wisconsin. The following excerpts from Sarah Watke's *Green Bay Press Gazette* article describe the goals of the Green Bay Surgical Center and how it would function in the delivery of ambulatory surgical services.

Center To Offer One-Day Surgery, By Sarah Watke, staff writer (January 1978)

Several Green Bay physicians today opened the first one-day surgical center in Wisconsin that is independent of a hospital. The Green Bay Surgical Center is located on third floor of the Medical Arts Building near Bellin and St. Vincent Hospital medical complex.

There are about 200 such centers in the nation including about five within Wisconsin hospitals. They are also called ambulatory, or "in-and-out" surgical centers. The centers provide operating rooms, recovery beds and emergency back-up for surgical procedures that don't require an overnight stay in the hospital. The operations can-

not be done in a doctor's office because they usually require general anesthesia.

The idea is to help hold down medical costs by eliminating unnecessary overnight stays in hospitals. Dr. Herbert Sandmire, one of four local developers, said the average patient and/or his insurance company will save "40 to 50 percent" of what the same operation would cost in a hospital. The center corporation will seek to meet expenses, but is not interested in making a large profit, he said.

The other physicians involved are Dr. Harold Hoops, a plastic surgeon, and Sandmire's gynecological associates, Dr. Drake Austin and Dr. Richard Bechtel. These four will be the original owners of the new corporation, "but it is anticipated others will become members," Sandmire said. Other physicians will be encouraged to use the center even if they are not members. Gynecological, orthopedic, urological and pediatric procedures are common at centers elsewhere.

Examples of some 20 typical procedures are tubal sterilizations, hernia repairs in children and adults, plastic surgery procedures, dilatation and curettage of the uterus, "myringotomy" on the ear drum, vasectomies and breast biopsies.. There are two operating rooms, a five-bed recovery area, recliner chairs, patient and professional changing rooms, and an instrument cleaning room.

"The surgical center has the same safety equipment as a hospital, such as cardiac monitors and defibrillators in case of anesthetic shock," Sandmire said.

Sandmire cited some of the reasons the center was established:
1) *The increasing cost of hospitalization. A tubal sterilization, for example, will cost a total of about $200 in the center compared with $300-$500 in a hospital (for a one or two night stay).*
2) *Improvement in anesthesia and surgical techniques making early release possible for 35 percent of all surgical patients.*

Sandmire cited some other advantages besides cost reduction:
3) *More effective use of doctors' and patients' time.*
4) *More personalized care than possible in a large departmentalized institution.*
5) *More privacy for patient.*

"The argument that surgical centers shouldn't be started where there are excess beds promotes the idea of putting a patient in a bed not because they need one, but because it is there," Sandmire said.

The surgical center was not subject to national health planning review because the cost of remodeling did not exceed $100,000, he explained. The project was also begun before a new state law made it reviewable as of July 1. "[the center] totally fits the guidelines of developing alternative, innovative methods to deliver care that are cost-containing without sacrificing quality," Sandmire said.

I presented a discussion of "A freestanding ambulatory surgical unit" at the 49th annual meeting of Central Association of Obstetricians and Gynecologists (CAOG) in Scottsdale, Arizona in October of 1981. I agreed with the author's conclusions that a freestanding ambulatory surgical center is cost effective, safe, convenient and well received by patients. My remarks were published in the June 1982 issue of *The American Journal of Obstetrics and Gynecology.*

Our early discharge program

Another innovation we developed in the late 1970s was to reduce healthcare costs with our early discharge program, which involved discharging patients within 24 to 36 hours of uncomplicated obstetrical deliveries. We arranged for a public health nurse to visit the patients' homes two to three days later. Our program preceded the widespread practice of shorter hospital stays by ten to fifteen years. I presented our experience with this program to the 1978 annual meeting of the Wisconsin Association of Perinatal Care.

Sexually-transmitted diseases conference

Another unanticipated reduction in health care costs resulted from our research indicating that married pregnant women do not need to be tested for gonorrhea.

In the fall of 1977, I was invited to participate in a two-day conference on sexually-transmitted diseases held at the Red Carpet Hotel in Milwaukee, Wisconsin. I reported on a study performed at our office involving 15,546 patients tested for gonorrhea, 1.8% of whom tested positive. Each patient was categorized as follows: having symptoms or a history of gonorrhea; sexually active unmarried; premarital exam; unmarried pregnant women; married pregnant women and miscellaneous.

It was interesting that, out of 650 premarital exams done during a five-year period, not one woman tested positive for gonorrhea. An additional finding was that among women who were pregnant, all of those who tested positive for gonorrhea were unmarried. This resulted in our discontinuation of gonorrhea testing for married pregnant patients. We did, however, continue testing unmarried, pregnant women.

This prompted our high school-aged daughter's French teacher, Ms. Tobias, to lodge a complaint against me before the State Medical Society of Wisconsin for discriminating against single, pregnant women. According to Ms. Tobias' complaint, we should have been required to either stop testing everyone - at great risk to our single, pregnant women - or test all married, pregnant women, which, because of the very low rate of positive tests, would be highly wasteful of health care dollars. In considering our choices, I could not help but remember the wisdom dished out by the famous bank robber, Willy Sutton, when asked why he robbed banks: he responded "Because, that's where the money is."

Our research findings guided us toward improved care at the lowest possible cost. Incidentally, I do not recall any problems resulting from Ms. Tobias filing her complaint against me with the State Medical Society of Wisconsin.

St. Mary's Hospital

Also weighing heavy on my mind during this time was an unnecessary plan to increase the number of hospital beds in Green Bay by 46 (at St. Mary's Hospital). November 9, 1977, 17 years after opening a new hospital on the West side of Green Bay, St. Mary's Hospital officials petitioned the Brown County Health Systems Advisory Committee for permission to build another new hospital with an additional 46 beds beyond the 134 beds already in existence. Meanwhile there were more than 180 unused beds available at the two East side Green Bay hospitals, Bellin Memorial Hospital and St. Vincent's Hospital.

As quoted in the *Green Bay Press Gazette* by reporter Sarah Watke, I spoke against the proposal:

> *Dr. Herbert Sandmire said it bothers him that supporters keep referring to a new hospital "for the West side. You'd begin to think it*

was 40 miles away. What decision is made is made for the city rather than for the West Side."

Referring to Dr. Bruce Stoehr's comment that the community needs a hospital on the West Side, Sandmire said, "The fact still has to be determined whether the community needs any more hospital beds." If beds are needed he said he would agree they should go to the West Side.

Sandmire also cautioned that physicians must be careful that they aren't protecting their own interests.

About one month later, the $20 million proposal was turned down by a 12 to 11 vote of the Northeast Wisconsin Health Systems Agency board. Interestingly, Bellin Hospital officials were asked if they would agree that there is a need for more beds in the community and whether they felt all three hospitals had been involved in planning this project. Spokesmen Donald Gaetz and Donald Wilson answered "no" to both questions. Michael Troyer, a University of Wisconsin- GB health economist, said that "Green Bay cannot afford to pay the cost of accessibility as presented by people who argue for the West Side." "We are all going to pay for them if there are excess beds built," he continued, "because of their impact on the other two hospitals."

Unfortunately, the Wisconsin Division of Health over-ruled the Northeast Wisconsin Health Systems Agency board, and the new hospital was built. Local and regional health planning agencies functioned admirably in the application process, but in the end it was political pull at the state level that ruled the day. My own position against the hospital expansion was based upon the anticipated higher health care costs generated by the wasteful spending of $20 million for the additional 46 unneeded beds.

Approximately ten months later, a *Green Bay Press Gazette* reporter wrote an article describing some difficulty the hospital was having in obtaining a low interest loan to finance the new hospital. She described opposition to the new hospital expressed by Council Member Annaliese Waggoner and by Dr. Jeremy Green, all of which was an example of "too little, too late," as by then the new hospital had been approved at the state level. As reported in the article:

Council Member Annaliese Waggoner of DePere said she didn't buy ideas that the West side is isolated from other hospitals, that private rooms are necessary, or that St. Mary's had cooperated enough with other hospitals.

Waggoner said Dr. Jeremy Green, chairmen of a cost containment committee for the Brown County Medical Society, convinced her that doctors will probably try to cut hospital use by 20-30 percent here and that Green Bay has too many beds, even though it has less [sic] per resident than most Wisconsin cities. Dr. Green recalled sharing these general ideas, although he said he had no specific information on the St. Mary's project.

At the time of the hearings, Dr. Herbert Sandmire of Green Bay was the only physician to publicly question the need. Green said if he'd been as informed then as he is since his appointment, he would have attended the hearings. He said he was skeptical then, but felt he shouldn't criticize because he didn't practice at St. Mary's. He said in general terms, the St. Mary's project adding 46 beds "is against everything I read."

Having spent my entire professional career in medicine, I'd be remiss not to reflect a bit on the current state of our nation's health care system, particularly at this critical time during which President Obama's health care reforms are slowly being implemented to bring down the sky-rocketing cost of health care in the U.S., which, in 2008, was $7000 per person.

It has always struck me that European health care is forty percent less costly than that in the U.S. but is of equal quality. There are many reasons for this stark difference between our country and European nations. The Europeans prioritize testing and treatments from most beneficial to least beneficial, and they eliminate payments for those which are the least effective. If this were tried in the U.S., we would have politicians and the public screaming that health care is being rationed and that individuals are being deprived. Furthermore, while the practice of so-called defensive medicine is commonplace in our country (with frequent use of medical tests and treatments to protect the physician from litigation rather than to provide true benefit for the patient), it is a much lower contributor to medical costs in Europe because of a different legal system that doesn't encourage frivolous lawsuits. As a result, European doctors pay lower rates for malpractice insurance and thus pass less of this cost on to their patients when setting their fees.

Americans, themselves, share some of the blame for the exorbitant cost of staying healthy as they flock to nutrition stores such as GNC to pay for large doses of vitamins and other supplements, despite there being no scientific evidence that such "megadosing" provides any health benefit.

Our unhealthy lifestyle choices do not help matters either. Twenty percent of U.S. adults and teenagers still smoke cigarettes; sixty years after it was determined that cigarette smoking is an extreme hazard to one's health. Our over-eating and general lack of exercise has contributed to our high rate of obesity, which has reached epidemic levels. The rates of both obesity, and its major complication, diabetes, have doubled in just the past 20 years.

Prescription drug costs have escalated as well. While our country develops 75 to 80 percent of the worlds new prescription drugs, many of these "new" drugs are not really new. Rather, they are of the "me too" variety, usually offering no improvement over the drugs they're designed to replace despite being more expensive than their predecessors. The way that these drugs are marketed has changed considerably over the past two decades, with the most significant change being the law that now allows pharmaceutical companies to market their prescription drugs directly to patients. The "Tell your doctor about it" commercials that are now commonplace on television and the internet lead to the overuse of the more expensive brand name drugs in place of the cheaper but chemically identical generic versions. Much of this reality is lost on the typical patient who shows up at the doctor's office with specific requests for "the medicine she/he saw on t.v.," thinking that this is the only path to better health. The busy doctor, in turn, often prescribes the more expensive drug to avoid angering the patient and to avoid the time it would take to have a thoughtful discussion about the equal efficacy of generic drugs.

In many ways, the costs of medical tests mirror the problems with prescription drugs. The explosion of media outlets over the past 20 years has completely transformed the way that patients get medical information. For example, while there are many reputable sites for medical information on the internet, such as WebMD, there are an equal number of sites that are not to be trusted as portals of valid, scientifically based information – and there is no filter for the patient to lead them to the correct information. The same can be said for the medical infomercials that Americans can tune in to on several of the 600 channels now available on cable television. It is hard to argue with a television expert about the need to megadose vitamin C when the typical viewer has very little scientific background to judge one way or the other.

The sensationalistic tendencies of many of our media outlets do not help matters either. When a newly touted drug or test has been shown by preliminary research to be effective, the news is on the front page, but when subsequent and more extensive studies disprove the drug's or test's benefits, the story is more often relegated to the back pages with smaller headline font. Furthermore, tests that may be more useful in the future management of patients are overzealously portrayed by the media. Recently, a test for Alzheimer's disease was approved by the Food and Drug Administration (FDA), and while this test might be useful in the research setting, it will initially provide very little direct benefit to patients. Nonetheless, if history is any judge, we can expect that, very soon if not already, this test will be demanded by elder patients and their families, and the cost of such testing will be distributed to all of the subscribers of these patients' health insurance plans. Even tests such as cholesterol levels, C-reactive protein, and prostate-specific antigen (PSA), while useful and important in the detection of those at risk for heart disease, stroke or prostate cancer, are ordered more frequently and more indiscriminately than is warranted by scientific evidence. A complete risk assessment carried out by the doctor, in conjunction with the patient, would help us limit the use of these screening tests to those cases where the risk profile makes the benefits of testing outweigh the costs of the test.

The creation of broad-based public and private health insurance plans over the past century, while making health care more affordable to the individual, has ironically driven up overall medical costs and made health care delivery more wasteful as well. When deciding to receive a given health care service, individuals do not realize that the costs, direct or indirect, are inevitably paid by someone. Instead, when a discussion of a certain test or treatment takes place between the physician and patient – especially concerning costs – the patient will all too often end the discussion by saying, "Oh, that's alright, I have insurance." Even the required deductibles that patients have to pay up front have been historically too low to influence what health care services they will receive. This system causes a substantial increase in health care services over what would be provided if each patient more directly bore the costs of care.

The problems of the third-party health insurance system are magnified at the end of one's life. The failure of many people to develop living wills stipulating desires regarding nutrition, intravenous fluids, cardiorespiratory support and other treatments leads to the common practice of prolonging death rather than meaningful life. Consequently, 40 percent of an individual's lifetime medical expenses are accrued in the last six months of life. And since these excessive costs are spread over hundreds of insurance prescribers, they are not as immediately felt by the individual. Instead, they are generally felt by the insurance plan's hundreds of subscribers who bear the brunt of escalating premiums and the general rise in price for medical tests and treatments. In September of 2010, I developed a sore inside of my lip. It was biopsied by the oral surgeon at a reasonable charge of $422, and the pathologist charged $183 to examine the tissue. However, Bellin Hospital entered an unbelievable $397 charge for a lab technician to prepare the slides for the pathologist – a symptom of a bigger problem.

While government-run Medicare and Medicaid have been modified over the years to cut out some of the wasteful practices, private insurers have lagged too far behind. The overhead expenses for private insurance in the United States are approximately 20 percent, compared to three to five percent for Medicare and Medicaid. So, why do my wife and I have no health insurance except for that required by law, that being Medicare Part A, which covers inpatient hospital care exceeding 24 hours in length? It is because, during the 51 years of my practice, I have witnessed how patients and their physicians waste health care resources. The individual choices about health care services provided are overly influenced by commercial insurance and Medicare/Medicaid considerations as opposed to considerations of the direct cost to the patient. This encourages the misconception that no one is really paying for those medical services.

My wife and I have decided not to participate in the wasteful pool which insurance coverage engenders and thus avoid Medicare Part B coverage. We are lucky, though, since we have been financially secure for most of our adult lives and are thus able to afford health care bills in the absence of a private insurance plan. However, most people are not in our financial situation, and the unfortunate irony of this is that those less fortunate individuals have no choice but to adopt a wasteful insurance plan since they could not risk having to pay catastrophic medical bills if something should happen to them – with the end result that our nation's health care costs continue to spiral upward.

CHAPTER 19

The picketers arrive

ON NOVEMBER 27, 1978, while I was in Iowa City giving a lecture at the University of Iowa's annual post-graduate course for obstetricians, I received a call from my office staff requesting advice on how they should respond to picketers who, for the first time, were marching around our six-story building. One suggestion by the office staff was to toss water balloons from our third floor window in an effort to wet down their enthusiasm. Rejecting that idea, I asked whether the protesters were young or old? "Old" was the response, whereupon I suggested that the staff should be courteous, friendly and non-confrontational. Thirty-three years later, that is still our policy, and the marching continues.

I did have one serious threat on my life, carried out by the boyfriend of a patient who had received an abortion. According to his family members, the boyfriend had purchased a gun for the purpose of shooting me, and they had notified the police of his actions. Going on 35 years now, he has not, thank goodness, carried out his plan. On another occasion, a bomb, determined later to be fake, was attached to the back door of our office building on a Tuesday night (the night of the week when I was on call and slept at our office).

As I write this book in 2010, I can report that six doctors have been assassinated by "pro-life wing-nuts" solely because they provided a legally sanctioned procedure. The last one, in 2010, was gunned down while attending Sunday morning church services.

The best way for me to describe the behavior and beliefs of the anti-choice crowd is to use excerpts from newspaper articles and their own words in letters to the editor where they provide "justification" for their actions. An example is a *News- Chronicle* article from January 24, 1990

110

under a large headline: **Anti-abortion sit-in by 106 at local clinic** by Nina Malmsten, *News-Chronicle* reporter. It is noteworthy that the *News- Chronicle* newspaper refers to anti-choice people as "anti-abortion," while the *Green Bay Press Gazette* calls them "pro-life." In my opinion the *News-Chronicle* "got it right." Excerpts from the *News-Chronicle* article follow:

Anti-abortion sit-in by 106 at local clinic

An anti-abortion sit-in at a Green Bay clinic ended peacefully Tuesday afternoon after five hours when protesters were told no abortions would be performed that day, an Operation Rescue spokeswoman said.

In a continuation of demonstrations throughout the country this week commemorating the 17th anniversary of the legalization of abortion, 106 protesters jammed the hallways of Ob-Gyn Associates of Green Bay Ltd.'s clinic said to perform abortions which is located in the Medical Arts Building at 704 S. Webster Ave.

While remaining peaceful, the group tried to prevent anybody from entering or leaving the clinic from about 8 a.m. to 1 p.m. sitting in a hallway after moving out of an elevator.

The protesters planned to stay at the clinic all day but after hour long negotiations between the group's leaders, and clinic representatives, decided to leave after being promised that no abortions would be performed at the clinic Tuesday, Lorri Fameree, a spokeswoman for the group, said.

No one was arrested because the clinic's doctors asked police not to intervene and the group remained calm, though officials asked the people to move outside.

The clinic had no comment on the issue.

"The clinic was closed today, that's what we wanted to gain," Fameree said, adding that the group would continue protesting as long as abortions were performed.

She said 106 people participated in the Tuesday occupation, with about 30 people coming from Chicago to protest, sing and pray, while 30 made the trip from Milwaukee and 20 from Upper Michigan, in addition to local participants.

Among the demonstrators Tuesday was Debby Fiala of De Pere, who described the protest as a "success."

"We wanted to show we as American citizens have the right to show that human beings, including unborn, have rights."

Examples of letters to the editors from writers who are against women assuming their reproductive rights are from the *Green Bay Press Gazette* January 30, 1990:

Ask the doctors

Here is a job for your investigative reporters. Find out why Drs. Sandmire, Bechtel and DeMott of Ob-Gyn Assoc. of Green Bay Ltd. allowed 106 pro-life rescuers to shut down their business on Jan. 23. Why didn't they call the police, as most businessmen no doubt would, and have these peaceful people arrested? Did the doctors have something to hide?

And while you're at it, find out why the Green Bay Press Gazette only reported the 50 pro-life prayer supporters who marched outside the Bellin Medical Arts building, and refused to report on the 106 pro-lifers who risked arrest on the inside. You might even ask the pro-lifers why they felt they should do such an odd thing. Hint: It has something to do with childkilling, and it is happening right here in Green Bay.

Kathleen S. Lawlor
233 Scout Way, De Pere, Wis.

Saw no coverage

Why was the lost lives of 25 million babies taken so lightly by the Green Bay Press Gazette?

Why wasn't the March for Life front page news? People have braved the cold to get across the point that 25 million babies have died in the past 17 years and many more will keep dying unless people take notice. How can they if there is no coverage?

Tell me, is a warehouse fire more important than 25 million babies? Is the local rent overcharge? Or maybe the man that paid his fine before name listing. Or BGH is safe for humans. This was front page news.

That is why this crime has been going on for 17 years. People won't take a stand because if and when they do, even the paper won't report it.

At the Medical Arts building, 147 people did a sit-in to block people from murdering their children. Apparently this also is not newsworthy material.

Betty Malcheski
County Road C
Green Bay, Wis.

Another view point was presented by E.L. Lee in his letter to the editor of January 29, 1990:

Protest gained no support

The recent demonstration of the pro-life advocates at a Green Bay clinic received substantial media attention. We saw coverage of peaceful picketing and passive occupation of entry and waiting areas. The more aggressive and abusive behavior was not displayed when the news media was present.

Patients and staff entering the building for 15 or more other offices were subjected to verbal abuse. Pregnant women and elderly people were pushed from elevators and forced to walk as many as six flights of stairs. Demonstrators forced entry and passage through a private office to gain access to a stairway where they again physically and verbally challenged those forced to walk up.

I understand the fervor of the pro-life cause. However, the end does not justify the means. Restricting the rights of others to health care and threatening the elderly and ill contradicts Christian behavior.

This aggressive demonstration did nothing to gain support for the pro-life cause among those who witnessed it.

E.L. Lee
704 S. Webster Ave.
Green Bay, Wis.

A letter supportive of Dr. DeMott appeared in the February 4, 1990 issue of the *Green Bay Press Gazette*:

Don't criticize doctors

In response to Betty Malcheski and Kathleen Lawlor letters on Jan 30, I have no respect for them or their organizations for pro-life.

My girlfriend and I, expecting our second child together, had an appointment on Jan 23 with Dr. Robert DeMott of OB-GYN Assoc. of Green Bay in the Medical Arts building. This day was the baby's due date, in for a final exam and check-up to see how things are going.

These people want to protect the unborn and save them. Well that day they neglected the unborn and turned her away from proper treatment and care. They would not let us off the elevator to get to our doctor's office. They had some unkind words to say about us and our doctor, and turned us away. Well they did not stop us. We saw our doctor that day and everything was fine.

On Jan. 28, during the Super Bowl, it is time. We called our doctor. He meets us at the hospital and at 6:24 p.m. he delivers a healthy baby girl.

We thank God for giving DeMott and his staff the ability and intelligence to be in such a field. We give them nothing but respect and praise for guiding us through two pregnancies and giving us two healthy babies.

The issue should not be against the doctors, but against the mothers. They are the ones making the decision to end life. The doctors are there for them, like they were for us guiding and giving proper care. Would you want these mothers to try and end life by themselves? I hope not, these unborn would suffer tremendously and who knows what would happen to the mothers.

Please point your energy and comments towards the mothers. The doctors are doing their jobs.

Matt Melum and Patti DeJardin
132 S. Chestnut
Green Bay, Wis.

The following February 5, 1990 letter supporting women's reproductive rights was received by the *Green Bay Press Gazette:*

Hits 'anti-choice' view

In response to letters supporting "anti-choice", especially K Lawlor's "Ask the doctor" (Forum, Jan 30), I would like to ask if these people would like all their rights taken away? They seem to have a very distorted view on freedom of choice. Take away a woman's right to have control over her own body and you leave the door open for all our rights to be abolished.

In China, the government dictates how many children a couple can have. The Soviet Union tells you where to live. Perhaps "anti-choice" would want to reside there, if they want the government to choose for them. These people seem confused. They say they abhor violence and yet they thrive on mayhem and disaster. These people attack people going into doctor's offices, they are constantly breaking the law and being arrested, and unbelievably they are proud of their barbaric tactics. They bomb clinics.

Pro-choicers are concerned with more than their own ideals, they are concerned with the welfare of the children already born into this world, children addicted to crack at birth, and the children who are physically and mentally abused, starving and living in poverty or worse, they are homeless. The little boy in Bob Greene's Jan. 17 article is a perfect example of child abuse.

But right to lifers don't mention the quality of life these little unwanted children have to endure. The anti-choice people are too busy trying to get their name or their picture in the paper for breaking the law.

I suggest anti-choice get off their self-righteous soap boxes and quit worrying if they are receiving enough press coverage and start taking care of the already thousands of unwanted children suffering in this country. Set up funds for them, quit trying to produce more of these unwanted, uncared for, underprivileged children.

Bobbie Peotter
812 S. Fisk
Green Bay, Wis.

A February 5, 1990 *Green Bay News-Chronicle* article reported on a Milwaukee abortion poll:

Poll finds majority favor abortion

Three out of five Wisconsin residents believe women should have the right to have an abortion, according to a statewide newspaper poll.

The Milwaukee Journal, *in its Sunday editions announced the results of its poll of 400 Wisconsin adults selected from a computer-generated random sample of telephone numbers. The poll had a five percent margin of error, the paper reported.*

A May 12, 1991 letter to the editor was headlined:

Grateful for doctors:

In response to Betty Malcheski's letter, May 2, concerning the doctors on the third floor of the Medical Arts building.

The right to an abortion is the law, Plain and simple. It is the law. Instead of condemning the doctors for part of their job description maybe Malcheski should talk to her congressman. She lives in a country where people have rights. Voice them against the law, not the doctors. They are only doing their job.

Because of one of those doctors Malcheski condemns, my husband and I have a perfectly normal 19-month-old-son.

*Because that doctor saw complications, my son is not handicapped.
She condemns this man, I thank God for Dr. DeMott. Our lives are
a little closer to perfect because of him.*

*And as for Malcheski asking the community not to "do business"
with the doctors in that building not only do we "do business" with the
doctors on third floor, we have a super family practitioner on the second floor. We would highly recommend any of the doctors in the Medical Arts Building. God bless the doctors.*
Tammy Ustianowski
1680 Cormier Road
Green Bay, Wis.

A letter to the *Green Bay Press Gazette* on April 3, 1992 was supportive of me:

Backs Sandmire as physician

*I cannot go without responding to a letter published recently cast-
ing aspersions upon a very good gynecologist, Dr. Herbert Sandmire.*

*Dr. Sandmire is a pillar of the community, involved in helping
women wherever he can; he is a sought-after expert in his field, the
care and science of women's illnesses.*

*When I go to Dr. Sandmire for care, in at times extremely diffi-
cult situations, his staff is kind and considerate. All doctors in the office
are prompt, respectful of their clients' own time and knowledgeable.*

*When we, the patients of OBGYN Associates or the Green Bay
Surgical Center, see Dr. Sandmire, we have confidence that we will be
cared for.*

*It makes no difference to me what goes on in any diagnostic room
between a woman and her doctor and I am proud to claim Dr. Sandmire as my physician.*
Beverly A. French
325 St. Francis Drive
Green Bay, Wis.

In the September 18, 1995 *Green Bay Press Gazette*, Sean Schultz
describes the emotions involved in choosing an abortion:

Choosing abortion an emotional decision

Different reactions for 2 area women
*At 16 years old, Shelly Banda had an abortion when she was told
it was her only option.*

Ann was 18 when she says she understood her options and decided abortion was the right choice.

Their experiences exemplify the debate over an abortion bill before the state Assembly. Should women know more when making a decision with lifelong impact? Or does a 24-hour waiting period create a barrier for women seeking a legal medical procedure?

Ann (not her real name), who wishes to remain anonymous, still says her only option 15 years ago was to end her pregnancy.

Banda says her abortion 22 years ago "was the worst mistake I ever made. I wish I had been stronger."

The emotion that accompanies most discussion about abortion will move to the legislative arena Thursday, when Assembly's 75 men and 24 women take up Assembly Bill 441. Among its provisions is a mandatory 24-hour wait before a woman has an abortion.

Ann, 33, had one when she was 18 and unmarried. While she regrets that she got pregnant, she says the abortion was the right choice.

The bill's 24-hour waiting period "treats women like children," she said. "I think they already have their minds made up before they go (for an abortion)."

In a companion article of the same date, Ms. Schultz reported on legislative activity and my testimony regarding the proposed bill:

"Coercing women," doctor says

Stalinism in the Wisconsin State Legislature?

A Green Bay obstetrician/gynecologist sees eerie signs of it in the abortion bill legislators are due to take up Thursday.

"Here the Legislature is coercing women," said Dr. Herbert Sandmire, adding that it is much like Stalin coerced those who disagreed with the state by forcing them into psychiatric hospitals.

Sandmire testified against Assembly Bill 441 at a July hearing in Madison.

Among other things, the bill calls for mandatory counseling by a physician for women contemplating an abortion and a 24-hour waiting period.

Sandmire said he testified "to try to prevent this intrusion into women's lives."

Sandmire said AB441 is "asking doctors at abortion clinics to try to talk women out of having abortions. What state interest is being improved by talking women out of abortions....?"

> *AB441 also is opposed by the State Medical Society of Wisconsin and the Wisconsin Society of Obstetrics and Gynecology.*
>
> *But Dorothy O'Malley, a co-founder of the Shield of Roses, a group that prays for an end to abortions, is all for the bill.*
>
> *Her group has marched outside the Medical Arts Building on South Webster Avenue on Wednesdays and Saturdays for nearly 18 years. That's where Sandmire's office is and where the group believes abortions are performed.*
>
> *"They're really not thinking clearly that it's human life," O'Malley said of women seeking abortions, "and someday they will regret it deeply."*

Unfortunately AB441 became law and provided another "hoop" women must jump through to exercise their legal right to have an abortion – a 24-hour waiting period between the initial consultation and returning for the abortion. This requirement meant that some patients, who may need to travel 200 plus miles to the abortion clinic, would need to stay overnight in the abortion clinic's city and be subjected to even more expense for no medical reason or benefit to anyone.

People often ask me, how do I put up with the verbal abuse heaped on me by the anti-choice crowd. My answer, first of all, is that they are expressing their constitutional first amendment right to free speech. Secondly, I learned an adage in first grade that I have subscribed to to this day, December 2, 2010: "Sticks and stones may break my bones but words will never hurt me." In addition, the anti-choice crowds have a very strongly held opinion that they are likely to carry to their graves. It would be futile to believe one could have a polite exchange of ideas with them.

CHAPTER 20

More publications

MY RESEARCH HAS always provided a welcome diversion from the political nature of the abortion debate, and in 1989 I authored an article entitled "Maternal mortality in Wisconsin: CVA (stroke)" in the *Wisconsin Medical Journal*. The focus of this study was to determine if women who were pregnant were at greater risk for having a fatal stroke than non-pregnant women of similar age. Using data collected by the Maternal Mortality Study Committee from 1971 to 1984, I reported on 20 pregnant women who had experienced a fatal stroke during or immediately after a pregnancy. Considering both the pregnancy-related and pregnancy-unrelated stroke deaths, the frequency of a fatal stroke in pregnant women (State of Wisconsin Health Statistics) is one per 49,039 births. This compares with one stroke death per 57,000 Wisconsin non-pregnant women aged 15 to 44 during a nine-month period.

Thus, pregnancy presents a relative risk for fatal stroke of only 1.16. These risk calculations suggest that only three of the 20 fatal stroke-associated maternal deaths were caused by the pregnancy. This study provided the first information indicating that the vast majority of stroke deaths occurring during pregnancy were not caused by, but were merely associated with pregnancy. Prior to the publication of this paper, maternal stroke deaths were routinely thought to be caused by the pregnancy.

I believe that the Wisconsin Maternal Mortality Study Committee, during its nearly 60–year existence, has been greatly under-appreciated. It has provided an important database, making studies like the one mentioned above possible. My own appointment to this committee in 1966 resulted in twice-yearly trips to Madison for the next 44 years and beyond to attend committee meetings, all at my own travel expense and with no remuneration. I was happy to do this, however, having always believed that the most satisfying activities are those for which we receive no pay. Furthermore, it is thanks to the efforts of organizations like the Maternal Mortality Study Committee that pregnancy-related maternal death rates have dropped from a tragic one out of 120 pregnant women in the 1920s to the current level of one in 7000 to 8000.

CHAPTER 21

Foreign friends

IN 1979 WE were invited to be part of the Wisconsin Medical Leaders Goodwill People-to-People delegation visiting Sweden, the Soviet Union and Switzerland, July 8th to 22nd. The People-to-People program was founded by President Eisenhower to foster a better understanding among people of the world. Our medical leaders' group was programmed to meet and exchange ideas with our counterparts in the countries visited.

At the dinner reception for group on July 11, Dr. Albert Chapman, Scientific Attaché at the U.S. Embassy, invited 14 Swedish physicians. We sat at a table with Dr. Bertil Hagstrom, his wife May and Dr. Chapman. It was by chance that we were seated with Dr. Hagstrom, a private practitioner (rare in Sweden) of gynecology at Sweden's only private hospital, the Sophiahemmet. He indicated that the government tolerates this 80-bed, private hospital simply to be able to better respond to criticism that Swedish citizens make about the lack of freedom in obtaining medical care. This hospital is primarily for gynecology, orthopedics and general surgery, particularly breast surgery. Patients utilizing this hospital must pay all of their hospital bills as well as the costs of participating in the social insurance plan. The patients who choose this private hospital are willing to pay their own bills when "free" care could be obtained in the social insurance hospitals either because they want their own doctor to take care of them, they believe private care is more efficient, or they wish to have a shorter waiting period for obtaining care. We had a great conversation with Dr. Bertil Hagstrom during which he invited us to tour his Sophiahemmet hospital and to visit with him and his wife at their home for cocktails prior to attending a reception which was given for embassy officials, the members of our group and a few Swedish physicians.

Our next meeting with the Hagstroms was in San Francisco during the meeting of the International Federation of Gynecology and Obstetrics in October of 1982. We enjoyed being seated with them at the meeting banquet and later joined them for a wonderful walking tour of San Francisco.

Our son Mike was on a low-budget tour of Europe which included a stop in Stockholm. The following post card sent to us April 26, 1983 describes a visit he had with the Hagstroms:

> *I just finished an incredible genuine Swedish meal cooked by none other than May Hagstrom and enjoyed also with her husband Bertil and daughter Maria. They took me out to an Italian friend's restaurant last night and I got to speak some Italian. I'm receiving the best hospitality to be found in Europe and probably the world!!! Your son, Mike.*

A day later we received a post card from the Hagstroms:

> *Hey there!!*
> *We are very glad to have the honour to have your son Mike here. We are talking of everything about our families and now we know everything about you!! Unfortunately Mike will leave us tomorrow again after 3 days in Stockholm. We love him already and hope that he will come back here for his honeymoon!! All the best to you From Bertil, May, Maria and Caroline.*

During the summer of 1986 from August third to the nineteenth, our family took a trip to Europe. Crystal and I, Cher and Tony, Yvonne, Mike and Dave went. Karen and Kevin were too involved in getting settled in their new home, Kev beginning a new medical practice at the West Side Clinic and Kev's studying for his specialty boards. We were sorry to leave them behind but hoped there would be another time when they could join a similar family trip. The trip was fabulous, seven of us together in a van driven mostly by Mike as he was more familiar with traveling in Europe. He had made the rule that each of us carry no more than a back pack and maybe a purse. As we checked into the Mainz Hotel, the porter was amazed by how little luggage we had for Americans. Traveling "light" turned out to be a good rule, and our family uses that rule whenever we can. We covered a lot of territory and had loads of fun.

Mike went the earliest, visiting friends in Italy. Next Yvonne and Dave went to Italy, joined Mike in Florence, and spent a week sightseeing. Those three then took a very scenic train ride from Italy through Switzerland, arriving in Lucerne on the first of August to a city-wide celebration of Swiss National Day, complete with people shooting fireworks out of hotel windows. Next, it was on to Frankfurt, Germany where they met the rest of us on the third of August. From there, we rented a van and headed to Mainz on the Rhine River to spend the first night together. With our able chauffeur Mike, we headed to Heidelberg the next day. The historic castle was first on the agenda, then old town, with lots of walking and sampling German food along the way. Antwerp was our next destination as we drove along the "Romantic Rhine Route" on the fifth to stay as guests of Dr. Arthur Van der Aa in West Malle, Belgium near Antwerp. He and his family had stayed with us when Yvonne's gymnastic club hosted the Belgian team here in Green Bay six years earlier. His two daughters were members of the Belgian team. We got to Dr. Van der Aa's about 7:45PM. Arthur had a girlfriend, Anita, at that time, which was good as he was not so lonely. According to our Yvonne, Arthur was just as nice as always. The children were great. Natalie was the oldest and would be going to medical school the next fall. Sabine was the next oldest, followed by son Guido, another daughter Muriel, and then his baby daughter, Sophie. We drank champagne and ate fancy crackers, cheese and chocolates. Then into the Jacuzzi and the indoor pool. We all agreed it was great to be there with these gracious Belgian hosts. We hoped they would visit us again someday. On the sixth, we woke up, had a dip in the pool and Jacuzzi, ate a huge breakfast, and rode into town with Arthur at 160 kilometers per hour (100 mph!). His Mercedes Benz was so quiet and smooth that it did not seem like we were traveling that fast.

We went to a cathedral and then to the Rubenshuis, or House of Rubens, the house and studio of 17th century Flemish painter Peter Paul Rubens, in Antwerp, where Cheryl had a field day with her camera, before we headed home for a Bar-B-Q, or should I say feast. We filled up on all kinds of veggies, soup, shrimp and salmon, and then realized that Arthur was still cooking chicken and steak on the grill. We ate meat with mushroom sauce that tasted like stroganoff, followed by ice cream with whipped cream, fruit, and of course chocolates.

We had a great time singing Flemish songs and talking and joking with the family. One memorable quote was Arthur's claim that "Giving up drinking, smoking and sex doesn't make you live longer, it just seems longer." The next day we woke up, had pannekoeken for breakfast, then drove to Knokke and rented a ten person pedal bike to ride up and down the board walk along the the "zee," or North Sea with four people pedaling and six riding. We walked to exquisite and expensive shoppes and devoured croissants with cappuccino. Later we drove to Brugge, a picturesque old town with canals and fancy lace stores.

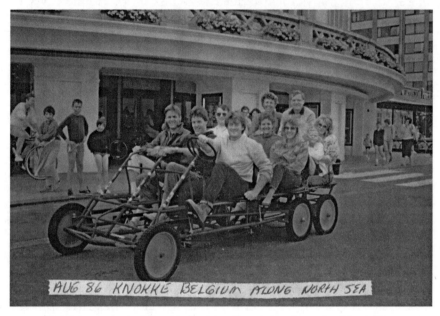

AUG 86 KNOKKE BELGIUM ALONG NORTH SEA

Sandmire travel clan with the Van Der Aas, along the North Sea in Knokke, Belgium. (1986)

The Van der Aa's house was big and beautiful, and we especially enjoyed the indoor swimming pool and outdoor jacuzzi. As our daughter Yvonne recalled, "One night, after my brother Mike sampled a little too much Belgian brew, he dumped an entire bottle of soap into the back yard jacuzzi (which Arthur pronounced Yah COO zee) and turned on the jets. Bubbles immediately began to rise out of the hot tub and eventually the entire yard was taken over by oozing foam about 5 feet high. We took photos of 'bubble people' and had a great time." Despite these misadventures, the Van der Aas treated our family like royalty and showed us much of Belgium, including the medieval town of Brugge, a coastal town of Knokke on the North Sea, and lots of pretty countryside. One night we had dinner at the home of Linda Sterkins, mother of one of the Belgian gymnasts who had stayed at our house on their Green Bay tour. It was the only thatched roof house we had ever been in. It was beautiful and we learned that homeowners insurance was more costly when you had a thatched roof due to the fire hazard. We said goodbye to the Van der Aa children but Arthur and Anita came with us to Zaandam for our first day there.

The Lammertsmas of Zaandam, Holland were another family that we valued as close and dear friends. Our daughter Cheryl was the first to make contact with them. As she recalled, "I first met Saskia and Agnes Lammertsma in Santa Barbara, CA in the late 70s. I was living with a friend of mine from high school in a big house near downtown. That summer she told me that the year before while she was traveling in Greece, she had met and gotten to know two sisters from Holland who were also traveling. The sisters were Agnes and Saskia Lammertsma and they were coming to Santa Barbara to visit. Then they were going to rent a car and spend the summer driving all the way across the U.S. seeing the whole country. To make a long story short, they arrived in Santa Barbara, we became fast friends and had so much fun together that they ended up staying with us in Santa Barbara the WHOLE summer, never seeing one other state! It was one of those summers that stays in your memory for a lifetime. Their nickname for me was "Cherie Baby," and now thirty-some years later, that is still what they call me. Fortunately for the Sandmires, through a lifelong series of visits back and forth to Europe by both families, we all got to know and love the delightful little family of Lammertmas, which also included the girls' parents Jack and Han."

In Zaandam, we were welcomed by Jack, Han, Agnes and her husband Robert. Cheryl was very happy to see Agnes and later Saskia again while the rest of us saw them as new-found friends. After soup and sandwiches, Jack took us on a boat tour down the Zaandam canals to Amsterdam, ending with dinner at an outdoor restaurant. Arthur and Anita had joined us for the first day and dined with us in Amsterdam before returning to their home. We saw lots of windmills and pretty country that did not look too different from Wisconsin.

When we returned to Jack and Han's house, Saskia took the kids out to where Julian's (her boyfriend) band was playing old rock and roll numbers. According to Yvonne, "they kept welcoming us and dedicating songs to their American friends. We tore up the place dancing. So we took over the floor when the band played. I think they thought we were a little crazy because we got into the music so much. Dave did his Egyptian dance and we all danced to the B-52's 'Rock Lobster,' the one where you go way down pointing at the floor. This Dutch guy started looking for what we were pointing at. We had the best time."

Sweetie and I slept in a room in their house while all of our kids slept on Jack's sail boat which was docked in their backyard on a canal.

Jack had recently retired as a teacher of auto mechanics in a technical school, so he took lots of time showing us around. We found the Europeans very warm, doing all they could to make our stay enjoyable.

The next day Jack took us on a boat tour of Marken Island, Holland before we drove on to Hamburg. After checking into our hotel the kids learned that it was the day of the Hamburg Wine Festival, so off they went by subway downtown, where streets were blocked off and everyone was partying. They saw a Renaissance play, ate at an outdoor restaurant where the waiter was tossing out toasted buns to the customers, and then danced to the music of a local rock-and-roll band.

From Hamburg, we were off again in a northward direction. Just before we got to the ferry to Denmark we drove to Priewall, a spot where you could park your car and walk 15-20 minutes to the East German Wall (actually it was a barbed wire fence). It was interesting to see the high fence, the East German soldiers, the watch tower and watch dogs. Immediately to our side of the fence was a nude beach, making the contrast of extreme freedom and no freedom <u>so</u> evident.

We took a ferry across the water to Denmark, and then drove on to Copenhagen, where we stayed in the top suite in the Kong Arthur Hotel with a good view of the city. That evening we all went to historic Tivoli, the second oldest amusement park in the world, with all kinds of restaurants, rides, games and fountains. Yvonne and Mike rode the roller coaster, Cheryl and Dave the Ferris wheel.

On the eleventh of August, we boarded another ferry to Sweden and then drove to our hotel in a very small town. Mike, Dave, Vonnie, Cher and Tony stayed in a little cabin out back of the hotel. According to them it was <u>very</u> rustic – maybe a little too rustic.

After breakfast in the hotel restaurant we drove the next day to Hovmantorp in Sweden's glass country, where we visited a glass blowing factory, Orrefors Crystal. We watched the hand-blown crystal being made and then bought some of their samples. The crystal means more to us after having observed it being made. The land in these northern European countries was very green and very clean. The coastal highway in Sweden looked much like our Door County in Wisconsin.

The drive to the large, old city of Stockholm took us through some beautiful farmland. The Swedish people were very nice, fairly conservative and kept everything neat and clean. We found our way to May and

Bertil Hagstroms' home, the friends we had met on a People-to-People tour in 1979. It's so nice having friends in Europe.

Dave, Mike and Yvonne stayed in the Hagstrom's home, while Tony and Cher, Sweetie and I stayed in a quaint pensione (bed and breakfast) just a few blocks away. That evening we met the Hagstroms' daughter Caroline and her fiancé, who is a dentist. Carolyn was in dental school at the time.

The next day we visited the old palace, formerly occupied by the King and Queen of Sweden, where we saw the crown jewels and tons of emeralds. Later that afternoon we went to an opera in the outdoor courtyard of another palace and almost froze to death. The blankets they handed out did little to keep us warm. At the opera we met Maria, the other Hagstrom daughter, and her boyfriend Per.

One night we had a Swedish Smorgasbord at a restaurant which had been in business since the 1700s. It was a spread of food like we had never seen. There were about 25 kinds of herring, plus everything else you could think of. Musicians strolled among the tables entertaining the diners. Very expensive!!

The next day we toured the palace where the current King and Queen reside and also saw a really old theatre and beautiful grounds with many sculptured hedges.

While shopping in downtown Stockholm, we bought Sweetie a silk blouse for her birthday and arranged for a cake. That evening at the Hagstroms, Bertil Bar-B-Q'd steaks, we sang Happy Birthday to Sweetie and then Bertil's brother and wife, daughter and a friend sang a Swedish birthday song. The Hagstroms presented the birthday girl with a porcelain flower vase made locally. We gave them the Indian weaving we had brought from home. We were treated to some beautiful music as all of their family members have beautiful voices and belong to a choir which commonly tours all over Europe.

After two full weeks of being pampered and gathering memories to last a lifetime, we headed home. We had seen and done a lot more in two weeks with the help of friends than we could have ever done on our own. No time was wasted wondering where to go and what to see. Except for Germany and Denmark, we had the help of our European friends in their countries.

In the spring of 1987, we were pleased to have Jack and Han Lammertsma visit us for a few days while they were traveling across our country in a motor home. We took them up to Door County and had lunch at Al Johnson's restaurant. We toured the Menomonie Indian Reservation and made a trip to Madison with them.

Later that summer Dr. Van der Aa and his wife Anita also spent a few days with us. We traveled to Door County but mostly entertained them in our home in Green Bay.

In 2002 we were again pleased to have Arthur and his new wife as visitors. We visited the Green Bay Packers Hall of Fame. Door County and Al Johnson's restaurant were again our destinations where Dr. Van der Aa fell in love with U.S. beef, having prime rib for lunch and again later that evening at a Green Bay restaurant.

We had offered the Hagstroms a complimentary two weeks at our Polo Beach Club condo which they finally accepted in the fall of 1991. Coincidentally, about that time we were returning from working on a legal case in Melbourne, Australia and had a stopover at our Polo Beach Club condo. We missed seeing the Hagstroms in our condo by only four days. Reviewing the pictures from the Hagstroms vacationing at the Polo Beach Club condo seemed strange, especially since we had just missed seeing them.

Our next connection with the Hagstrom family was during our attendance at an American College of Obstetricians and Gynecologists (ACOG) District II meeting held in St. Petersburg, Russia and Stockholm, Sweden in October of 1996. We were very happy to renew our friendship with them, and they were excited to see us.

We received permission to invite them to the October seventh ACOG buffet dinner in the Stockholm City Hall, the site of the Nobel Prize awards ceremony. In addition, we invited them to attend the farewell function with us. To see another part of Sweden, our Medical and Scientific session members were bused for one day to nearby Uppsala, another beautiful city.

Bertil and May Hagstrom wrote to us prior to our arrival in Stockholm:

> *Stockholm, 9/19/96*
> *Dear Chris [sic] and Herb Sandmire!*
> *We are very happy for and see forward your arrival to Stockholm 5 Oct. We will contact you at the Sheraton Hotel Saturday evening for discussion of the schedule for the following days. We are very happy for your invitation for us to attend the reception in City Hall evening, Monday 7 and the Farewell function evening Wednesday 9. We also like you to meet us in our home and other get together possibilities with our family.*
> *At the moment now we are healthy and wish you to very welcome to Stockholm and to us!*
> *Sincerely, May and Bertil Hagstrom*

Following our return home to Green Bay, We wrote to our Swedish friends expressing our appreciation for the incredible time we had in Stockholm especially the dinners at the Drama Theatre Restaurant, daughter Maria's home, and finally at their home.

The Van der Aas and Lammertsmas had another opportunity to host members our family the following year when our son Michael and his wife Lisa visited Belgium and Holland in September of 1997. Both of these families had also visited our children living out West on trips to the United States.

In March of 1998 Jack and Han Lammertsma joined us for a three-week stay in our Maui Kamaole condominium. The thing I remember most was that Jack had a digital camera which we were not familiar with at the time. My wife remembers how they taught her how to poach salmon to bring out its best flavor. It was nice having them with us as we got to revisit all of the usual Maui sites: Iao Needle, Hana, the drive around the island, whale watching with Bruce Morse, the Haleakala Crater, and the Winery. One evening we splurged on a dinner at Sea Watch and went "slumming" one afternoon at the Polo Beach Club pool.

On June 18, 2006, at the conclusion of our Rhine River cruise, the Lammertsmas met us at our ship,the "Rembrandt," in Amsterdam, and accompanied us on a canal tour of the city. We saw the house where Anne Frank wrote her diary, followed by lunch on the waterfront. We had lots of catching up to do as we had not seen them in eight years.

Unfortunately both Jack and Han passed away in 2010 within a few months of one another. We felt fortunate that we had the chance to spend some time with them in 2006 while they were still in relatively good health. They are gone now, but will live forever in our memories of Europe.

CHAPTER 22

My medical legal experience

IN THE FALL of 1981, my professional responsibilities expanded to include being an expert witness in liability cases involving lawsuits filed against nurses and physicians. In my first case I was asked to testify on behalf of one of my Green Bay colleagues, Dr. John Utrie, who was being sued by Milwaukee attorney James Murphy.

Although unknown to me at the time, this was to be the first of 451 legal cases which I would participate in over the next 30 years. Of these, I provided depositions for 145 cases and trial testimony for 62 cases. All told, I found no evidence of negligence (i.e., malpractice) in 80 to 90 percent of the cases, and, in those instances, I agreed to help defend the nurse or physician as an expert witness. Five to 10 percent of the cases I reviewed between 1981 and 2001 came from plaintiff attorneys, and I found that I could support the plaintiff's position about 10 percent of the time. Beginning in the late 1990s, my publication emphasis shifted to shoulder dystocia and brachial plexus injury, and thereafter most of the cases I reviewed dealt with those issues, with my giving testimony almost exclusively on behalf of the health care personnel with emphasis on causation.

The role of the expert witness is to interpret and explain medical issues and facts which the lay person would not likely understand and to define the prevailing standards of care. The expert must determine whether those standards have been violated, and whether the care in question caused the patient's injury.

Wisconsin Jury instructions by the judge

The Wisconsin civil justice system defines medical negligence in the following manner:

In the care of his/her patient the doctor was required to use the degree of care, skill, and judgment which reasonable doctors would exercise in the same or similar circumstances, having due regard for the state of medical science at that time. A doctor who fails to conform to this standard is negligent. The burden is on the plaintiff to prove that the doctor was negligent.

A doctor is not negligent, however, for failing to use the highest degree of care, skill and judgment or solely because a bad result may have followed his/her treatment. The standard you must apply in determining if the doctor was negligent is whether the doctor failed to use the degree of care, skill, and judgment which reasonable doctors would exercise given the state of medical knowledge at the time of the treatment.

You have heard testimony during this trial from doctors who have testified as expert witnesses. The reason for this is because the degree of care, skill and judgment which a reasonable doctor would exercise is not a matter within the common knowledge of lay persons. This standard is within the special knowledge of experts in the field of medicine and can only be established by the testimony of those experts. You, therefore, may not speculate or guess what the standard of care, skill and judgment is in deciding this case but rather must attempt to determine it from the expert testimony that you heard during this trial.

The cause question asks whether there was a causal connection between negligence on the part of the doctor and the plaintiff's injury. A person's negligence is a cause of plaintiff's injury if the negligence was a substantial factor in producing the present condition of the plaintiff's health.

A doctor has the duty to provide the patient with information necessary to enable the patient to make an informed decision about a treatment and alternative choices for treatment. If the doctor fails to perform this duty, he/she is negligent.

To meet this duty to inform his/her patient, the doctor must provide the patient with information a reasonable person in the patient's position would regard as significant when deciding to accept or reject the medical treatment. In answering this question, you should determine what a reasonable person in the patient's position would want to know in consenting to or rejecting a medical treatment.

My concepts of the duties of the expert witness

From the perspective of the expert witness, it is important to understand that the jurors will remember and carry more perceptions than remembered factual information into the deliberation room. What characteristics does the expert need in order to provide memorable perceptions? Well, the expert must know all of the facts and issues in the case. She should be perceived to be knowledgeable and competent. Likeability is a very important characteristic. He should be the kind of doctor that individual jury members would like for their personal physician. The expert should project humility, but not at the expense of competence. The effective witness is polite, even with the opposing attorney and especially with the judge. The expert should use humor cautiously, and usually it should be self-directed.

In conveying facts to the jury, the expert should use language that is understood by a lay person. The testimony she gives should be presented in a slow, deliberate and memorable fashion. The expert should maintain eye contact with jurors to determine their degree of understanding of what the expert is saying. The expert should remember that courtroom trials provide a certain amount of stress to all of the participants, including the jurors.

While the legal definition of an expert witness requires only that he possess a medical degree, the medical definition of an expert entails someone who has demonstrated expertise "in the issues which are in dispute," as evidenced by his research, presentations, publications, and teaching positions. Defense expert witnesses are more likely to fit the medical definition than plaintiff expert witnesses. In fact, in a study entitled "Characteristics of Physicians Who Frequently Act as Expert Witnesses in Neurologic Birth Injury Litigation," published in the August 2006 issue of *Obstetrics and Gynecology*, Harvard researchers Aaron Kesselheim and David Studdert reported that plaintiffs' frequent testifiers were older (on average, 57.2 compared with 50.8 years), less likely to have subspecialty board certification (38% compared with 95%), and had fewer academic publications (5.0, on average, compared with 53.5) than defendants' expert witnesses. Kesselheim and Studdert concluded that "plaintiff witnesses have fewer markers of expertise than defendant witnesses."

Amazingly, and unfortunately, plaintiff's "expert" witnesses generally have not demonstrated medical expertise regarding the issues for which they are providing testimony. That is, they generally have not performed research, published articles in peer reviewed journals on any subject, or held teaching appointments. Having no publications on any subject, they cannot be confronted by the defense attorney with inconsistencies between their trial testimony and previous publications.

In my first case, the jury ruled in favor of the obstetrician, Dr. Utrie, apparently because others and I provided believable testimony.

They found that the obstetrician did everything he was supposed to do despite the poor outcome. In this case, there were two large law firms representing the obstetrician and hospital, respectively, and therefore I was asked soon thereafter to participate in numerous other cases. In the 1980s most of these cases were from Wisconsin, but beginning in the late 1980s and early 1990s, because of my publications, I began to receive out-of-state cases.

In the fall of 1988, the late Paul Grimstad, an excellent defense attorney, asked me to assist with the defense of my partner, Richard Bechtel, by serving as an expert witness. Attorney Grimstad reasoned that my extensive knowledge of the literature and my ability to talk to jurors in layman's language more than offset the potential perception of bias which jurors may have. He was right, in that the jurors found no causal negligence and no money was paid.

On May 10, 1995, at Attorney Grimstad's request, I again testified on behalf of Dr. Bechtel. This law suit demonstrates that good doctors, if outcome is poor, are as likely to be sued as not-so-good doctors. Dr. Bechtel was one of the most competent, caring, dedicated obstetrician I have known. The only good news is that we achieved a defense verdict again with my participation as a defense expert witness in both of these cases – an exceedingly satisfying experience for me.

In this latter trial, it was understandable that plaintiff attorney Cates would try to plant the seeds of bias in the jurors' thinking as demonstrated by his following questions (Q) and my answers (A).

Q. Now, the other thing is, which is obvious, you are Dr. Bechtel's partner?

A. Absolutely.

Q. And you work at St. Vincent?

A. Yes. Yes, sir.

Q. Work with the nurses?

A. Fight with them too.

Q. I believe that, but you work with the nurses?

A. Yes, sir.

Q. And in fact, you have the same insurance company as the hospital, do you not?

A. I don't know that.

Q. Do you know who your underlying insurance carrier is?

A. Yes, sir, I do.

Q. And can you tell me who that is?

A. Yes, the state plan.

Q. And it's the same as Dr. Bechtel's?

A. Yes, sir that I know.

Q. And whatever happens here obviously can have some input on that, can it not?

Mr. Grimstad: I am going to object to the relevancy of this line of questioning.

The Court: He may go a little further.

Q. What happens in this case could have an impact on some publicity in regard to your clinic, correct?

A. I don't think it would be, should we say, clinically significant.

Q. Sure. You can use any word you want, Doctor.

A. I don't think it would be practically significant. I don't think Dr. Bechtel would be judged on that basis. I don't think our clinic would be judged on that basis.

Q. At least you would hope not, correct, Sir?

A. I really hadn't even thought about it. You have.

Next, Attorney Cates didn't help himself by picking a fight with me over hypoxic-ischemic encephalopathy versus neonatal encephalopathy terminology:

Q. On page 704 of that particular exhibit, the author states "Hypoxic-ischemic encephalopathy is the term used to designate the clinical and neuropathologic findings of an encephalopathy that occurs in the full-term infant who has experienced a significant episode of intrapartum asphyxia." Did you know he talks about that?

A. Oh, I know, but I think the preferred term now is neonatal encephalopathy without, in the term, trying to suggest causation when there are multiple causes for encephalopathy, so I think he is using the term hypoxic-ischemic encephalopathy in a non-modern way.

Q. Do you think the Dr. Volpe, which is I believe..... I think he.... this is... Exhibit 60, this is a part of his 1995 Year Book that goes from page 211 to 369 where he talks about hypoxic-ischemic encephalopathy. Do you think that he is using a term that is not modern?

A. I believe that, yes. I think that's the modern....the researchers are saying now that sometimes when you use terms, it presents a barrier to really searching more closely for the true cause and that generally we don't in our diagnosis include what we speculate is the cause of that diagnosis. I think I said one time, it is like a dog chasing its tail.

Q. I know you said that.

A. You don't need .... to look for the cause because it's incorporated in the definition, but it should be labeled neonatal encephalopathy rather than coming to premature conclusions about the cause and actually putting that in the definition or the name of the problem. I have looked through, and many people are using neonatal encephalopathy because they've been mistaken in the past, that it wasn't hypoxia in a normal baby coming into labor in a normal fashion.

Q. Doctor, Did you bring in any literature that you put on the board here that used the term neonatal encephalopathy?

A. I think I read it. Maybe it was in your literature but, yes.

Q. Do you recall any up on the board.... we are going to go through here, so if you see any words neonatal encephalopathy, stop me and point that out, OK?

A. I will. I will certainly do that. I think it was in your literature though.

Twenty four pages later Attorney Cates, while reading to me from a treatise, which included neonatal encephalopathy:

Q. OK. And then we are going to take a look at the next blow-up which is plaintiff treatise number 24, the Gaffney article. What you didn't read or tell the jury was this paragraph (neonatal encephalopathy)?

A. There it is. Neonatal encephalopathy. You asked me to point it out to you.

Q. Thank you.

A. Thank you for helping me help you.

Many physicians owe a debt of gratitude to the late Paul Grimstad, Dr. Bechtel's attorney, who I believe was the best defense attorney in Wisconsin. I had the privilege of working with him on 20 cases without a single loss. He described his work with me on those cases in his letter to Ms. Peterson supporting my nomination for the Wisconsin Medical Alumni Ralph Hawley Distinguished Service Award.

Nash, Spindler, Grimstad & McCracken LLP
Ms. Karen S. Peterson, Executive Director
Wisconsin Medical Alumni Assoc.

RE: Dr. Herb Sandmire
Dear Ms. Peterson:
As an attorney who represents physicians and hospitals in medical negligence actions, I have had the pleasure of working with Dr. Sandmire on

numerous cases over the last 25 years. Dr. Sandmire's contribution to the defense of these cases has been immeasurable. No matter how busy he might have been, Dr. Sandmire never refused a request to review a chart. His work was prompt, thorough and insightful.

If Dr. Sandmire felt the care fell below the applicable standard he would say so. If, however, he felt the care should be defended, he would work tirelessly with us to make sure that we presented the most effective possible defense.

Dr. Sandmire's encyclopedic knowledge of the obstetrical and gynecological literature is truly impressive. The opinions he advanced were always well thought out and completely supported by the literature. When he was called upon to testify he did so candidly and the opinions he offered were well supported. He was always able to effectively defend his position.

It has truly been a pleasure working with Dr. Sandmire as we defended medical negligence cases. Our success rate in cases in which he was involved was extraordinarily high. The obstetricians and gynecologists practicing in Wisconsin owe Dr. Sandmire a tremendous debt of gratitude. I am pleased to submit this letter in support of his nomination for the Wisconsin Medical Alumni Association Ralph Hawley Distinguished Service Award.

Very truly yours,
Paul H. Grimstad

Attorney Grimstad was also helpful in defending my former partner, the late Dr. Austin, in a lawsuit filed by Dr. Austin's former "friend" Attorney Robert Schaefer. My letter to Attorney Grimstad thanking him for his efforts follows:

Ob-Gyn Associates of Green Bay
704 South Webster Ave.
Green Bay, WI 54301

October 31, 1991
Paul H. Grimstad
NASH, SPINDLER, DEAN & GRIMSTAD
Manitowoc, WI 54220-2992
Re: Jorgenson vs. Austin

Dear Mr. Grimstad,
Thank you for all of your attention directed toward defending the name and reputation of my late partner Stephen Drake Austin. I

have reviewed your correspondence with Atty. R. W. Schaefer dated October 18, 1991 via fax.

Atty. Schaefer's assertion that Dr. Austin withheld information regrding his health status is particularly troublesome. In fact Dr. Austin had no symptoms or physical signs of cancer until sometime following the surgery in question. In view of the fact that Atty. Schaefer knew Dr. Austin to be an outstanding member of the medical profession and the Green Bay community, his inane allegation is further perplexing.

Finally, Atty. Schaefer has identified certain unspecified attitude problems that I have which he thought would be corrected by the aging process. The said attitude problem is Atty. Schaefer's explanation for our refusing to settle this meritless claim. Actually, defending the good name of one of the finest persons I have ever known requires no special motivating factors. Whatever else I may have lost by the ravages of the aging process, my sense of smell remains intact.

Thanks again for all of your diligent assistance in resolving this matter.

Sincerely,
Herbert F. Sandmire M.D.
Cc: Mr. R. W. Schaefer
Mr. Brian R. Mudd
Mr. Donald M. Rouch
Mrs. Stephen D. Austin

Support of my fellow obstetricians and family physicians in the medical legal arena by functioning as an expert witness has been a big part of my non-patient care activity along with teaching and research. In order to prevent possible personal bias I am going to rely on the letters from defendant physicians and their attorneys with whom I have worked to describe any contributions I may have made in their defense.

9/25/93
Dear Herb,
I want you to know I appreciate your coming to Madison to witness on behalf of the defense the other day. Your words of wisdom were well-spoken. Your experience was made obvious by your statements. Your affirmations were succinct and true by every measure known to me.

Thank you so very much,
Sincerely, Walt Schotten (Beloit, WI obstetrician)

Elm Avenue Clinic, S. C.
Waupun, WI 53963
January 24, 1994

Re: Chavis Sheriff Case
Dear Dr. Sandmire,
Thank you for the support and expertise you provided us for the defense of our malpractice case.

The argument provided by our expert witnesses was enough for the jury to decide in our favor after a very short deliberation.

Litigation was such a stressful experience for both of us. I hope we can overcome this without any negative feelings to our career, work and attitude to patients.

We appreciate all the help you provided our lawyer, Mr. Nick Meeuwsen.

Sincerely, E. G. Arellano, MD and C.P. Arellano, MD

Menn, Nelson, Sharratt, Teetaert & Beisenstein, Ltd.
Appleton, Wisconsin 54912-0785

March 25, 1982
Re: Brenda Lindloff vs. Lakeview Medical Center
Dear Dr. Sandmire:
I have just received word from the Panel that they found that both the hospital and the doctor were not negligent in any respect. I think in large part that this was obviously due to your outstanding efforts. I would assume that the claimant will not take this case to the Circuit Court.

Thank you so much again for your efforts, which have been greatly appreciated by both me and the hospital. I look forward to work with you again.

Very truly yours, Jonathan M. Menn

Attorney at Law
500 West Madison Street
Chicago, Illinois 60661-8000
September 25, 1997

Re: Ketura Pace, a minor, through her Mother, Tabitha Pace-Mitchell v Dr. Vanko and Nurse Bauman
Dear Dr. Sandmire,
I am very pleased to enclose a copy of Judge Kowalski's order of September 24, 1997 entering judgment in favor of Dr. Vanko and

against the plaintiffs. He granted our post-trial motion for judgment notwithstanding the verdict. It was his impression there was no evidence upon which the jury could have found in favor of the plaintiff.

This will effectively end this case. Again, we sincerely appreciate the benefit of your time and expertise. Needless to say, Dr. Vanko was ultimately very happy with the way things turned out. Thanks again for all your help.

Very truly yours, BOLLINGER, RUBERRY & GARVEY, David R. Barry, Jr.

This is an example of a rare occurrence with the Judge overruling the jury verdict.

RE: Stafford. 8/26/2004. email from me to Attorney Renee B. Crawford

Dear Renee,

We arrived home this afternoon. Hope the trial is still going well. Regarding the final arguments I would recommend that you use the blowup of the 14 mostly university centers, to illustrate not only the non-shoulder dystocia brachial plexus injuries, but also to emphasize that all of these centers, and you can list the numbers, do indeed have many cases of Erb's palsy. You recall me saying that all of these university centers are still searching for a way to prevent Erb's palsy. Was Dr. Tyler expected to succeed while the major university centers in the country have not? I think this is the most important thing for the jury to realize before their deliberations begin.

Sincerely, Herb S.

Re: Stafford trial. 8/28/2004.email from attorney Renee Crawford to me

Dear Dr. Sandmire,

I am thrilled to let you know that we won the case The jury was out for about an hour and 15 minutes on Friday afternoon and came back with a defense verdict at about 4:20. Of course, Dr. Tyler and Dr. Holt were thrilled and so very relieved. Your testimony was the key to the whole case, of course. You gave the jury the explanation for what happened, and I used the doll and the pelvis in my closing argument to make the point again and again that Dr. Tyler did not cause the injury by use of excessive traction. We talked to only a couple of jurors afterward and learned that they were with us fairly early on (they did not think much of Mrs. Stafford) but that your testimony about the cause of the injury was crucial to the defense. They loved you and found you extremely credible, likeable and knowledgeable. No surprise there! We will talk with more jurors and I will give you more feedback then.

Thanks you so much for all your incredible help with this case. I truly could not have done it without you, and only you. You helped me to understand this case more than any witness/expert I have had in any case ever, and I cannot thank you enough for your detailed attention to everything, your unwavering support and, of course, your famous flexibility!! (the time of my testimony was scheduled and rescheduled and scheduled and rescheduled and finally scheduled and actually took place)

It was truly an honor and a pleasure to work with you and to meet you. It has been one of the best things about this case, in addition to getting to know Dr. Tyler and Dr. Holt and Dr. Cefalo. I will never forget what you did for me and for these physicians. Please give Mrs. Sandmire my fondest wishes. And please send your invoice to me right away. I will be in touch soon with additional juror feedback.

With warmest regards, Renee

I received a letter from one of the defendant doctors, Michael J. Tyler, written September 15, 2004. His letter describes the emotions that most physicians have when charged with malpractice. After all, doctors are to help and not hurt patients!

Dear Dr. Sandmire,

It's taken me a little time for the confusing mixture of feelings that follow the favorable verdict, but now I'd like to thank you for your effort on our behalf. I can't tell you how much I appreciate your diligence, your patience and your dedication to our case. Even more importantly, though, was your belief in us as physicians at a time when we began to question ourselves.

I am not an "old man" when it comes to time in practice, but I do feel very old when it comes to practicing in the current medical legal environment. The past three years have taken their toll on me in my profession and personal life and I'm really questioning whether I want to be practicing medicine three years from now. Coming out of this trial, I am feeling a need to communicate to my patients and patients-at-large, how this changes one in terms of their approach to practice and ability to practice.

Lastly, Dr. Sandmire, I would like to say that I respect you not only for the questions you asked that led to a better understanding of

Erb's palsy, but also as a role model for myself and other physicians. Your belief (evidenced by your lifetime commitment) that a physician is not only a practitioner but also an educator of patients, students, and fellow physicians is one that we can truly look up to in times where our every motivation is called into question.

With heartfelt gratitude, Sincerely, Michael J. Tyler

Sweetie has been my constant companion and helpmate during the past 30 plus years by attending all the trials, always sitting in the back row. I have previously suggested she might be breaking the law by signaling whether I am doing well or not so well by her facial expressions. She denies it. After the Stafford trial was over and we had the news of the defense verdict from Attorney Crawford she (Sweetie) sent her following reflections to our children byemail.

8/29/04

Good Morning,

We are finally getting a little caught up after being gone for 10 days. As you know, we went first to Corinne's in Lilesville and had a nice but short visit with her. Then we headed to Raleigh where Dad was to meet with the attorney on Thursday evening and testify on Friday morning. Well, it kept getting pushed back by half days or whole days and he finally got on the stand on Tuesday at 11 AM. They did not get finished with him until 11 AM on Wednesday. We were housed in a nice LaQuinta motel in a nice area while waiting for Dad to testify. So we used their pool and Jacuzzi, got a lot of reading done, did a lot of walking around the area and even did some shopping in a huge Prime Outlet across the highway.

I will copy to the end of this email, an email we just got from Renee Crawford, the defense attorney (a little bragging). All of our waiting around, putting up with delays etc. was evidently appreciated and worthwhile. Dad kept telling Renee that we were flexible. She kept apologizing for all the delays. I told Dad that Renee, the two doctors being sued and another expert witness Dr. Cefalo, (Chrm, Dept. of OB/Gyn, Univ N. Carolina and editor of the OB/GYN Survey Journal) all acted like Dad was a legend. I guess he is. We had dinner with all of them one night at a neat French Restaurant.

Peterson, Johnson & Murray, S.C.
Milwaukee, Wisconsin 53202-4767

October 23, 1996
Re: Gainer v Sturino, et al
Dear Dr. Sandmire
The Supreme Court has refused to accept the Gainer's petition to review the decision of the appellate court affirming the trial court's dismissal of the Gainer action. In short, the defense has won. This means there is nothing further for any of us to do on this case. If you still have any records that relate to this case they may be thrown away.

The Sturinos, the Petersons, and the Ratzels, Mary Lee is my partner, will be at the OB conference in Puerto Rico in January. If you and Mrs. Sandmire will be in attendance, we must get together to celebrate. (We did.)

Very truly yours, Donald R. Peterson

The defense verdict which we received from the jury was appealed to the Appellate Court. The basis was my testimony to the jury that I was obligated to pay my daily liability insurance cost of $270 while testifying in court and while not seeing a single patient that day. Plaintiff attorney presented arguments that the jurors' knowledge of that information would prejudice them away from a plaintiff verdict.

The Appellate Court affirmed the trial court's dismissal of the Gainer action. The attorney for Gainer appealed the Appellate court's ruling to the Wisconsin Supreme Court which declined to review the Appellate Court's ruling. "In short, the defense has won."

North Shore Medical Clinic
Sturgeon Bay, WI 54235-1495
April 6, 1989

Dear Herb,
I am a little tardy in doing so, but I do wish to write you a few words of appreciation for your help during my recent malpractice case. Due primarily to your deposition and that of Dr. Harry Farb, the plaintiffs' attorney, advised the patient that she would probably lose at trial and be forced to appeal, which, as you know, prompted them to ask for dismissal.

I want you to know how much this meant to me, Thank you!
Sincerely, Richard C. Murray, M.D

Moser and Marsalek, P.C
St. Louis MO. 63102-2730
May 16, 2002

In re: Logan Miller, Minor v Associates in Women's Healthcare
and William Scott Magill, D.O.
Dear Dr. Sandmire:
It goes without saying that you were extremely helpful in our defense. The voluminous materials that you supplied to me were invaluable to me in preparation for the cross-examination of Dr. Edelberg and Mr. Allen and in preparing for my opening statements and examinations of you, Dr. Moore and Dr. Magill. Your testimony was stated with confidence and authority, yet not so rigidly as to suggest bias.

Although Dr. Magill stated that excessive force was not used, we had to overcome the dogmatic views of Dr. Edelberg, Mr. Allen and some of the literature. I think clearly the articles that you have written as well as some of the other articles by your colleagues overcame the rigid presumption by Dr. Edelberg. In my opinion, Dr. Edelberg did not perform well in his cross-examination in accusing you and others of trying to cover up physicians' negligence by writing these various articles.

If you have any further questions about the trial or your testimony, please give me a call. Many thanks for your assistance.
Yours truly, Peter F. Spataro

Nash, Spindler, Dean and Grimstad
Manitowoc, Wisconsin 54220-2992

March 10, 1994
RE: Sheffer v Myers, MD
Dear Dr. Sandmire:
I am pleased to advise you that the jury found no negligence on the part of Dr. Myers. In fact, the deliberations lasted approximately 15 minutes. The manner in which the jury dispatched the plaintiff's case is directly attributable to the quality of expert testimony presented to them. On behalf of Dr. Myers and myself, thank you for your assistance in this case. You did an excellent job.
Very truly yours, William R. Wick

Attorneys at Law
Eau Claire WI 54702 0390

August 14, 1992
RE: Claimant: Lisa Robinson
Dear Dr. Sandmire,
We are very pleased to enclose a copy of Judge Peterson's Decision finding that neither Dr. Stenzel nor Dr. Burgess was negligent. The Decision is carefully organized and well-reasoned. I believe it will stand up on appeal.

On behalf of Dr. Stenzel, I would like to thank you for your time and effort in defense of the care provided by the doctors. Your testimony was certainly instrumental in obtaining this decision.
Sincerely, Thomas J Misfeldt

Nash, Spindler, Dean & Grimstad
Manitowoc, Wisconsin 54220-2992

November 4, 1991
Re: Megan Suring v Clyde Siefert MD
Dear Dr. Sandmire:
I am pleased to inform you that the jury found Dr. Siefert was not negligent in the above-captioned action. This verdict was due in large measure to your willingness to assist us and the excellent testimony you gave at the time of trial. This case could not have been successfully defended without your assistance. On behalf of Dr. Siefert and myself, please accept our appreciation and sincere thanks.

It is only through the involvement of highly respected individuals such as yourself that justice can truly be accomplished in cases of this type. Your willingness to become involved is greatly appreciated. I hope, should the occasion arise in the future, that I can call upon you again to provide an objective analysis in a matter in which our law firm is involved.

It was a pleasure to work with you. Again, on behalf of Dr. Siefert and myself thank you for all of your efforts.
Sincerely yours, William R. Wick

Schober, Ulatowski & Hinchey S.C.
Green Bay, WI 54301-1069

September 25, 1987
Re: Cota v St. Mary's Hospital
Dear Dr. Sandmire:
*James J Hinchey, Jr. would like to thank you for your cooperation
and assistance in the Cota case. Your time and knowledge assisted in
our successful defense on behalf of Dr. Gallagher. We could not have
been as successful without your assistance. Thank you.*
*Very truly yours, Maureen Vogel, paralegal for James J Hinchey,
Jr.*

Menn, Nelson, Sharratt, Teetaert & Beisenstein, Ltd.
Appleton, Wisconsin 54912-6631
Re: Parisi v Methodist Hospital

January 30, 1989
Dear Dr. Sandmire:
*As you by now know, we have won a total victory in the above
case. In fact, the judge directed a verdict in our favor on the creden-
tialing claim after the close of all the evidence, which means that he
found as a matter of law that there was nothing to that claim. The
jury then found 12-0 in favor of Dr. Anderson on the claim that he
was negligence, thus resulting in a total victory for all of the defendants.*

*I think your testimony was instrumental in the very successful
result we achieved in this case. I certainly appreciate again the opportunity I had to work with you, your suggestions and your analysis of
the case.*

Thank you again for your assistance.
Very truly yours, Jonathan M. Menn

Hoffman, Hart & Wagner LLP
Portland, OR 97205

December 19, 2000
Re: Ricker v Kaiser
Dear Dr. Sandmire:
*As I trust you have heard by now, the jury deliberated for six
hours and found in Kaiser's favor on every aspect of our case. Your case
preparation and very effective trial testimony were pivotal insofar as*

our success and I wanted to thank you on behalf of Dr. Friedman and myself.

I hope your holidays are the very best they can be.

Best personal regards, John E. Hart

Sager, Colwin, Pavlick & Associates SC
Fond du Lac, Wisconsin

January 30, 2001
Re: Cody Alt v Charles J Green MD et al
Dear Dr. Sandmire:

I know I personally spoke with you after the trial. I was very pleased with your help and careful review of the rather complicated issues in this case. Obviously the jury appreciated the input and time spent by virtue of its no negligence verdict. (I am of the opinion as well that the issues that we dealt with on causation were just as instrumental in helping the jury more easily come to its conclusion on negligence, even though they didn't have to decide a "causation question.")

My personal best to you and I look forward to working with you in the future on other cases.

Very truly yours, Steven P. Sager

Dellington@bjpc.com

3/15/2007
Re: Courtroom impressions in Hinton v Ferris
Dear Attorney Ellington,

A note from Dr. Sandmire returning to Maui: I observed some smirks and suppressed laughter from four or five jurors during my cross examination and therefore in my opinion we can't lose. The worst that can happen is a hung jury.

Sincerely, Herb Sandmire MD

Brown & James, PC
St. Louis, MO 63101-2000

Re: Hinton v Ferris
March 16, 2007
Dr. Sandmire:

I am pleased to report that the jury returned a defense verdict after 15 minutes of deliberations. The jury found your opinions to be well reasoned. They resented Miller "beating up on you". We appreciate your time and expertise. Please send your statement for payment. Early next week I will be sending your pelvic model, doll and DVD.

Thank you, David P. Ellington

Hoffman, Hart & Wagner
Portland, OR 97205

August 10, 2007
Re: Warling trial
Dear Dr. Sandmire:
I wanted to let you know John and Kelly received a defense verdict last night. The judge spoke with the jurors right after the verdict was received. The judge then relayed some of the comments to the attorneys. You will be happy to know that the jury indicated that the top three doctors (out of all the experts that testified) they believed and liked were: Dr. Depp, Dr. Sandmire and Dr. Connor. We really appreciate your help.

Thank you, Melissa Jorgenson, Assistant to John E. Hart

Dr. John S Honish
Oconto, WI 54153

November 3, 2004
Dear Dr. Sandmire,
I just had my annual exam with your son, Kevin, today. He asked how I was doing, when was I thinking about retiring, etc. I told him I was doing much better since my malpractice lawsuit was dismissed in April of this year.

The whole discussion I had with Kevin was therapeutic – I just don't discuss it with many people. I told him I was initially angry, anxious and depressed. I told him that I contacted you and you were very kind, helpful and gave me almost an hour of your time.

My attorney, Paul Grimstad & Associates, moved for dismissal and finally in April of this year the judge granted it with absolutely no payment and no chance for the plaintiff to refile. She had 45 days to appeal, but we never heard another word from her.

Kevin tells me that you have talked to several doctors with similar problems in the past. I want you to know it's very comforting and very helpful. I called your home initially and spoke with your wife when I was trying to reach you. She was also kind and helpful, please give her my "thanks".

I want to thank you from the bottom of my heart. You are a rock and a real credit to your profession.
Sincerely, John S. Honish, MD

The email below is my response to Attorney Grass's staff phone call notifying me that the plaintiff's attorney had dismissed the Lopez v Coy case and also asking me to review the medical records in the Bridges v Coy case.

April 5, 2010 1:46 pm
Re: Lopez v Coy

Dear Attorney Grass,
Congratulations on obtaining the dismissal of the Lopez v Coy claim. Also, since I am going to be 81 years old on 4/09/10, I have decided not to take any more new cases. I highly recommend my "young" partner, Dr. Robert DeMott.
You were kind to assume that my being an expert "had much to do with their dismissal decision."
I will forward your Bridges v Coy letter to Dr. DeMott as well as your email regarding the achievement of a dismissal in the Lopez v Coy case.
I have enjoyed working with you and meeting you in my office in December 2009 during which time I believe I introduced you to Dr. DeMott.
Sincerely, Herb Sandmire MD

jeff@davis-grass.com

April 5, 2010, 4:07 pm
Re: Lopez v Coy
Thank you Dr. Sandmire. Thank you also for the referral to Dr. DeMott. I did meet him at your office. You were kind enough to introduce him to me when I was there in December. I am sorry you are not taking more cases and am sorry we did not have a chance to do a trial together. As for the plaintiffs in the Lopez matter, the attorney for the plaintiffs was really irate the day he received our designation of experts and specifically mentioned your name when I saw him later that day for a deposition. As such, there is no doubt your stature in the field was significant in the decision to dismiss the case. Finally, thank you for all you taught me in those three hours we were together when I met you at your office last December.
Jeff Grass

Mock trial

The following telephone conversation was taped May 1, 1997 to be included in a mock trial presented at the 17th Annual Berlin Memorial Hospital Summer Conference July 31, August 1 and 2, 1997.

Attorney James Doyle/Dr. Herbert F. Sandmire telephone conversation, May 1, 1997

Dr. S. Hello

Att. Doyle: Good Morning

Dr. S. Well, good morning Jim. I didn't want to bother you, but I just had a few curiosity questions.

Atty. Doyle. All right. You did get the message from my secretary.

Dr. S. Yes, in fact that was called in at 11AM

Atty. Doyle. They didn't get the verdict until 8:30

Dr. S. And that's one of my curiosity questions. I know we had seen Stan Graven there Wednesday morning in the restaurant and we knew he was on. Was he the last witness?

Atty. Doyle. He was the last witness on Wednesday, the last live witness, then they read some more depositions. We had our jury instruction conference and our final arguments about 2:30 in the afternoon, didn't finish until after 5:30. And then the jury was given the option of either staying or coming back the next morning. They opted to come back the next morning. They started deliberating at 8:30 and at 9:30 had a verdict.

Dr. S. Well they're very efficient.

Att. Doyle. (laughing) I said to my son Jamie who was there as we were coming back in, I said "If we lost this case, we really got hammered,"

Dr. S. Yes. (laughing)

Atty. Doyle. Because how could we, they couldn't have, you know, found the damage in that length of time. But they found no negligence on either doctor. They found no conscious pain and suffering on the child and they determined that the damages were zero because the instruction, and I was careful to point out to them, if you only give damages for the negligent conduct of the doctor and if you find the doctor isn't negligent the answer is zero.

So, but I wanted to again thank you Dr. Sandmire. I have told people who ask about the trial, but particularly those that knew about you, I think you were absolutely the cornerstone to the victory. And the reason I say that is, that everything that you had to say you backed up with some article. It wasn't just a matter of "hey I'm looking at the same monitor strips and I can see something different than somebody else." You know we had them every place that we touched base "here is what the articles you have published have said on the topic." So, I was very impressed with that.

One of the things that I said to the jury in my closing argument was, "you know Mr. Egan tried to attack Dr. Sandmire collaterally by saying he testified and he's got 6 cabinets or 5 cabinets full of depositions," I said "But understand, he keeps his depositions because he is consistent." He doesn't have to worry about having other people say "well here he said one thing and here he is saying another thing." He says the same thing, and so he is consistent, and if they had anything at all to impeach him on, they would have done it without just telling you about 6 cabinets full because they could have looked at all of his depositions and found something different if there was any inconsistency."

Dr. S. Yes, Egan set that up for you. (laughing)

Atty. Doyle. (laughing) So, you know all that collateral bullshit if they have something to say that any point that you said was wrong. They should tell that to the jury. And so I think that's when the case was decided. I think Graven did a commendable job. But, we could have dispensed with that and argued when you were done.

Dr. S. That brings up my question. See, I thought that trial probably wouldn't be over until next week but you must have moved right along and when did Farb testify?

Atty. Doyle. We cancelled him.

Dr. S. Oh, he was supposed to come after...

Atty. Doyle. He was supposed to come Thursday morning and we pulled the plug on him. Read parts of his deposition. Cuz, you know, he couldn't have said it better than you and I said "Hey, all he can do is hurt us."

Dr. S. Well, I agree with you. But I didn't know that, but what he might have testified ahead of me, I didn't know that....

Atty. Doyle. No, he was going to come in Thursday morning and we pulled the plug on him and we threw out McDonald, just read a little bit from McDonald's deposition and that was it.

Dr. S. Well okay. I won't hold you up any more.

Atty. Doyle. All right. I appreciated all your help, you knew the case, you knew the authorities, you were just great. And you have a great style with the jury. So we may meet again Herbert, we may meet again.

Dr. S. I told you I would have the jurors laughing. And I said don't worry about it even though I didn't know what it would be. But I did have them laughing, didn't I?

Atty. Doyle. You did.

Dr. S. And then, once I know they're laughing, they're going to listen to me.

Atty. Doyle. That's right. You gotta make the best impression. All right. Well I will send you Barness' deposition and send me your bill because this outfit they throw nickels around like they're man hole covers and they take a while to pay bills.

Dr. S. Which outfit is it?

Atty. Doyle. Physicians Insurance Company of Wisconsin.

Dr. S. Okay, well I'll send the bill in promptly.

Atty. Doyle. All right.

Dr. S. All right.

Atty. Doyle. Sure Herb.

Dr. S. Thank you.

Doyle. Bye.

Dr. S. Bye.

Unless you, as a physician, have been sued it is not possible to know the agony, stretched over five years, until you have an opportunity to have your day in court. You will be confronted with exaggerated statements in "the complaint" which do not relate to what actually took place in your care of the patient. You will be advised to not discuss the case with anyone and so you suffer in silence. You begin to lose confidence in your ability as a physician. Not uncommonly, mild depression sets in accompanied by sleepless nights. You will be exposed to untruthful statements during the deposition and trial testimony by plaintiffs' "experts" who have done no research or published articles relating to the issues in the law suit. One might ask, why they do it (provide untruthful testimony) and the answer seems to be to attract more cases to review and get paid from other plaintiffs' attorneys.

As one can imagine, following a defense verdict the accused physician experiences monumental relief and is highly appreciative of any contribution I have made to the "successful" outcome. Actually, the physician, by winning protects his/her reputation but at the costs of five years of agony, countless hours in preparing for deposition and trial and two to three weeks out of his/her practice for attendance at the trial.

Interestingly, on February 8, 2011, Bill Wick, partner with the late Attorney Grimstad and an attorney I had worked with on a few cases, called and asked me to review an alleged misreading of a fetal monitor strip case. I told him that I had stopped taking new cases over a year ago, that I will be 82 years old in two months and that, with the long time – up to six years – it takes for cases to come to trial, it would be unfair to the defendant doctor for me to function as an expert witness in the defense of the claim.

I will admit that it was quite flattering to hear him practically beg me to participate in his defense of the female obstetrician practicing in near- by Appleton. He, Attorney Wick, believed that being local and having a national and international reputation would be exceedingly helpful in persuading the jury to the defense point of view in the claim especially being venued in near-by Appleton.

Sweetie, who could hear the conversation on the speaker phone, thought that I was about, at one point, ready to "give in" and agree to work to help defend the claim – but I didn't.

CHAPTER 23

Teaching family practice residents

IN 1979, THE University of Wisconsin-Madison Family Practice residency program was in need of more obstetrics hands-on training for their residents. They asked me to develop and become medical director of an Advanced Obstetrics Rotation in Green Bay. Each of their 14 third-year residents would spend two months in the Green Bay obstetrics rotation. My Green Bay obstetrics colleagues and I agreed, and the next year the program began. I received a joint appointment as a clinical assistant professor in the University Departments of Family Medicine and Practice and Obstetrics and Gynecology. Subsequently, I was promoted to Associate Professor in 1983 and to Professor in 1986.

The program gradually expanded to involve other University of Wisconsin Family Practice programs in Appleton, Wausau and Eau Claire, as well as to provide training for residents from the freestanding Marquette, Michigan program. As our program became known across the nation, we occasionally accepted residents from residency training programs outside of Wisconsin.

My teaching involved meeting with the residents for one hour each morning for discussion of didactic obstetrics subjects. With the onset of my teaching responsibilities, I began to accumulate important research articles concerning 18 separate obstetrics topics, collating them in binders by topic groups. The binders were available to the residents and served as a basis for one of the residents to lead a discussion at each of our morning meetings. Examples of obstetrics topics discussed were non-progressive labor, fetal heart rate monitoring, breech presentation, forceps and vacuum-assisted delivery, low birth weight, hypertensive disorders of pregnancy, cerebral palsy, diabetic pregnancies, epidural anesthesia, macrosomia, shoulder dystocia, brachial plexus injury, twins, and ante-partum testing.

After the first three or four years of our residency program, I began to remove from the binders one article for each one added. This was done in December of each year, with the quality of the added article weighed against the quality of an article already being used. The articles I selected came from the three or four journals that I perused on a regular basis. At the end of each of the two months rotation, I told the departing residents that they knew more obstetrics now than they would ever know in the future. Though we didn't call it this at the time, we were developing a training program centered on the principles of evidence-based practice.

Green Bay Press Gazette reporter Peg Schmeling described the beginning of the Green Bay Advanced Obstetrics Rotation in her 1980 article as follows:

> *Almost every morning at 6:30 a.m. Dr. Nancy Scattergood and Dr. Richard Barad meet to exchange information about patients.*
>
> *One is going on hospital duty for 24 hours; the other is off for 24 hours.*
>
> *Such meetings aren't unusual for doctors. But, in this case the two doctors are married to each other and this is the way they've been seeing each other for the last couple of months.*
>
> *Scattergood and Barad are in their third year of residency at the University of Wisconsin-Madison They are the first to come to Green Bay for a new post-graduate obstetrical training program for residents in family practice.*
>
> *As such, they've been assisting local doctors with their patients at St. Vincent and Bellin Memorial hospitals since Nov. 3. They will be leaving Tuesday.*
>
> *It's been a hectic time for them – long working hours and little time together. But, they agree, it's been worth the sleepless nights and 24-hour duty stints.*
>
> *We see each other to go on rounds and pass the beeper," Barad quipped. "And every two weeks we get to spend a couple of days together."*
>
> *Each has participated in the delivery of about 150 babies. They've become familiar with the many different complications which can occur during delivery, and how they are handled.*
>
> *Each will be 29 when they finish their three-year residencies at the UW Medical School in June. They met while students at the*

Albert Einstein College of Medicine in New York City. They are from different small towns in New Jersey.

In Madison, physicians are used to working with residents because there are so many of them there. But this is the first time such a program has been introduced to Green Bay's physicians.

They worked with 14 obstetricians and about 12 family doctors. "We see a lot of different practice styles." Barad said. "There are a lot of different ways of doing things. So we can pick and choose the ones we want."

Dr. Herbert Sandmire, coordinator for the training program, said the UW asked the Green Bay hospitals to affiliate with its medical school "because of their recognition of the excellent medical care provided in the Green Bay community. They wanted to have their residents working in an environment where they could obtain the best experiences."

Plans are for two residents to come to Green Bay every two months to work with local doctors in obstetrics.

Unsolicited feedback is probably the most reliable means of measuring one's teaching effectiveness. I much appreciated the following very nice letter from Lauren Fuller and Jim Harrison, married residents who also participated in our residency program. The letter follows:

1-02-84

Dear Dr. Sandmire,

Hello and Happy New Year! Lauren and I just wanted to drop you this note to let you know how much we appreciate all that you did for us. It seemed kind of soapy to tell you in person but we thought you should hear it one way or another.

We are indebted to you for a number of things. As coordinator of the residents, you do a good job at a task that is vital to us but that probably no one else wants to do. The time that you spent with us was way above and beyond any obligation. You allowed us goodly amounts of participation in the delivery room. You taught us things about obstetrics we didn't know and didn't know we didn't know. You imparted a very pleasant atmosphere into the field of obstetrics. But we think your most important lessons, and the ones we are indebted to you most for were to question the rules and that there is a lot of flexibility in obstetrical management. They may sound like obvious lessons for a physician but they aren't, particularly in the field of obstetrics. To see someone practicing those principles (which neither of us had seen prior to Green Bay was very worthwhile).

For all those things, thank you very much,
Sincerely, Jim Harrison and Lauren Fuller

As I reread Jim and Lauren's letter, I reflected on the almost unbelievable number of morning meetings with the residents that I have attended during the 29 years as the medical director. The calculations: 52 weeks minus five weeks (vacations/medical meetings) = 47 weeks x five days = 235 meetings per year x 29 years = 6,815 hours, all as an uncompensated volunteer.

During 1986 the UW residents, as a way of showing their appreciation, awarded me with the First Annual Clinical Teaching Award presented by the graduating family practice resident physicians at the University of Wisconsin Medical Center "in recognition of valuable contributions to the education of resident physicians."

Additional teaching awards followed:

> *2000. Community Physician Teaching Award: Fox Valley Family Practice Physicians; University of Wisconsin Family Practice Residency recognizes Herbert F. Sandmire M.D. for his Compassionate and Skillful Care of Patients and his Enthusiasm, Dedication and Skill in Teaching Resident Physicians.*
>
> *2008. "Each year the graduating class of the Marquette Family Medicine Residency Program selects a physician who has provided them with outstanding outpatient teaching during the course of their training. I am pleased to inform you that the graduating residents have selected you as the recipient of the "Senior Outpatient Award." This award honors your teaching of outpatient knowledge and skills to our residents."*

Amazingly, the awards seem to be coming for my doing what I'm supposed to do!!!

[The advanced obstetric residency program is still ongoing. I met with Missy Simon, a third-year resident from the Madison program, on May 26, 2010, my last day of practice with Ob-Gyn Associates of Green Bay.

The whole purpose for teaching is to expand the effect of your ideas beyond what would otherwise occur. This is the primary motivating factor for most teachers. How can what I teach students, physicians or others help their future patients? The qualities that make a teacher very good include the willingness to take the time to prepare and become the best teacher possible. It requires a genuine interest in making your pupils better. It requires knowledge of what your pupils do not know. It requires knowledge of what they need to know. It requires the presen-

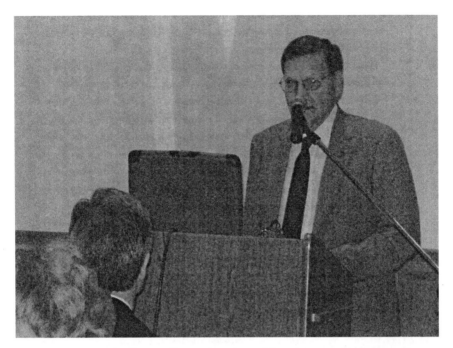

Receiving the 2008 Senior Outpatient Award from the graduating residents,
Marquette, Michigan

tation of what they need to know that is useful in the care of their future
patients, in an interesting, memorable fashion. An observation I made
early in my career was that teaching, research and patient care are three
individual activities, each of which complement the other two. Teaching may also expose that which the teacher does not know!

Benefits of teaching include the positive feedback from those who are
learning. It provides reassuring information that the teacher's time is well
spent, is providing sound information, and is appreciated. Included below
is a small sampling of the letters from additional residents expressing their
appreciation for their obstetrical experience in Green Bay:

Alleghany Family Physicians of Altoona, Pennsylvania Hospital

Family Medicine Residency Program
September 12, 1995
Dear Dr. Sandmire:
Thank you for writing the letter of recommendation for my priv-
ileges at Altoona Hospital. By receiving such privileges, it has
prompted a review of our Obstetrical/Family Practice Priveleging

System, and I was appointed to [the] Ad Hoc Committee so that we can have the Family Practitioners and Obstetricians in the Community working in closer communication.

Your teaching methods have been so exceptional, that I clearly remember my Green Bay Rotation and the terrific morning lectures which prompted critical thinking in Obstetrics. I am in charge of our Obstetrical Curriculum in the residency and I am also the Program Director for the Family Practice Residency Program. Thus, I feel that it is critical to my success as one of the many teachers of the obstetrical issues of the residents, that I obtain copies of the series of binders that you send to Fellows for the Fellowship Program. I would like information on how I can obtain these, and the cost.

You have been the strongest influence in my career regarding obstetrics, and I am happy to say that six years out of my Family Practice Residency training, I am still delivering low-risk obstetrical patients, and plan to continue to do so for the duration of my career. Your articles on Fetal Monitoring have prompted much stimulating discussion throughout my years with Obstetricians, and other Family Practitioners, Residents, and Medical Students. I would like to thank you once again for the excellent education which you and your fellow Obstetricians provided for me during the time of three months that I spent at Green Bay in 1986 and again in 1989.

Sincerely and With Best Wishes in Your Ongoing and Successful Career

Elissa J. Palmer, M.D.
Program Director

Appleton Family Health Center
229 S. Morrison St.
Appleton, WI 54911
Dear Dr. Sandmire,

Thank you for the update of the OB topics for the Ringbooks. I always look forward to their arrival.

In the past year, we have revised several things in our OB curriculum, including making the ring notebooks more accessible to the residents. Instead of being kept in the library where we thought they were safer and could be controlled easier, they are in the residents' call room. Every resident is made aware of the contents, with a bibliography and are encouraged to review them while they are on the OB rotation.

You provide a very valuable service to our residents and our training program with these updates. Thank you for your efforts!!

Congratulations on your award for Outstanding Wisconsin Obstetrician-Gynecologist. I can't think of one more deserving of the honor.
Sincerely,
John N. Allhiser, MD

A Note: Your thoughtfulness is truly appreciated
I hope you have some idea how much your generosity in time and teaching has impacted us. Thank you so much. We hope you continue to enjoy teaching for years to come so that many other students of medicine can benefit from your knowledge! Have a great summer.
Respectfully, Kris, Bob, Jewel

Family Practice Residency Program
Asheville, North Carolina
Dear Drs. Bechtel, Cavanaugh, DeMott and Sandmire
Greetings from Asheville, North Carolina, where the rhododendrons are in bloom. I want to thank you for being so supportive of my OB experience in Green Bay during March. It was an excellent opportunity to see and participate in a different style of obstetric care. It was refreshing to see so many normal deliveries and women deliver "naturally." I learned a lot from all of you and appreciate your willingness to involve me in the care of your patients and your willingness to teach. The morning sessions with Dr. Sandmire were particularly memorable and have inspired me to continue pursuing evidence-based obstetrical care. I have recommended an OB rotation in Green Bay to my colleagues, so you may see some Panther fans trickling up there. I hope you will be able to give them as warm a Packer welcome as you gave me, but I doubt you could match the 18 inches of snowfall in 24 hours. I hope to see you all again when I return to Green Bay visiting family. Good luck in hiring another physician to add to your very special group. Thanks again.
In peace and health,
Lisa Lichtig, M.D. (daughter of Joanne Hanaway and the late Attorney General Don Hanaway

Family Care Doctors, Marquette General Hospital
June 11, 1993
Dear Dr. Sandmire,
I would like to thank you for the opportunity I had over the last couple of months to work with you and others at Bellin and St. Vincent's Hospitals. I found it to be a great learning experience. I did

appreciate the one on one teaching that you especially gave during my time spent there. I would also have to single out Doctors DeMott, Bechtel, Scheckler and Steve Sehring for their time that they spent with me as well as teaching and during deliveries.

I am enclosing a paper that states how many deliveries I had obtained during my two months in Green Bay. I did obtain 70 deliveries and I will outline exactly how many vacuum extractions, third degrees, etc. that I also was able to participate in as well. This may be needed in my attempt to obtain low risk obstetrical practices at Grandview Hospital in Ironwood, Michigan. I will send an envelope with my Hurley, Wisconsin address on it so that you can return it to me in the event that it is needed.

I would once again like to thank you for the time you spent with me. I found it to be probably the best experience throughout my three years of family practice residency. I would highly recommend the obstetrical elective rotation to any other of the residents here in Marquette.

Sincerely yours, Tod C. Lewis M.D.

Wausau Family Practice Center
995 Campus Dr. Wausau, WI 54401

May 5, 1995
Dear Herb,
Mark Reuter, M.D. returned several days ago from his rotation with you. He was full of enthusiasm and praise for the rotation. Enclosed is a copy of his evaluation form for your feedback.

I reviewed the evaluations of the other seventeen residents that I know of who had spent time on the OB rotation with you and found some definite consistent threads. They were unanimous in how useful and excellent the experience was. They found your academic approach to the literature to be very insightful and liked the volume and variety of procedures to which they were exposed.

On behalf of the residency I want to thank you for all the time and attention you have put in on their behalf. I know how much I enjoyed the two weeks I spent with you on my mini-fellowship prior to coming to Wausau and am very mindful of how much I learned during that refresher course.

Two of our residents, Alison Dalrymple and Rick Mayrer, are presently on rotation with you. I think you will find them to be extremely conscientious, knowledgeable, and eager to learn. I hope you will enjoy them as much as I have enjoyed them the past two and one-half years.

Since January I have been Associate Director of the Wausau residency. I have a rather interesting combination of teaching, administration, and patient care. I enjoy supervising the residents with their obstetrical experiences. I do a small volume of OB care myself as well.

Thanks again, Herb, for all your help over the years.

With warmest personal regards, Glen Heinzl, M.D.

Duluth Clinic
400 East Third St. Duluth, MN 55805

January 15, 1996

Dear Dr. Sandmire,

We have been practicing family medicine for a little over a year in International Falls, Minnesota, a town of 8,500. The OB experience we received in Green Bay at Bellin and St. Vincent's Hospital has been enormously helpful in our clinical practices. We feel comfortable in obstetrics despite being 100 miles from the nearest obstetrician. You provide a valuable learning experience and I hope you will be able to continue to provide residents with the much needed learning opportunity that is unique in Green Bay.

Please share our thanks with your colleagues and feel free to share this letter with hospital personnel. Thank you again.

Sincerely, Kristin K. Elliott, M.D., Randall O. Card, M.D.

"Can Community docs do research for the sake of it?"

Family Medical Center
Paudre Valley Hospital
1025 Pennock Place
Fort Collins, CO 80524-3998
August 1998
Greetings,

I wanted to write to thank you for sharing your time and patients with me. I had a great experience in Green Bay.

One of our faculty obstetricians and I were talking about the rotation. He asked "what's in it for them?" and didn't quite seem to believe that community docs would teach and do research for the sake of it. Well, I sure do appreciate that you do!

Thanks,
Kristen Dhen

CHAPTER 24

Mini-fellowship program

LESS THAN A year after the residency rotation was established, five University of Wisconsin family practice faculty members, having received feedback from the residents, came to Green Bay to update their obstetric skills. This led Dr. Tom Meyer, Director of Continuing Medical Education (CME) at the University of Wisconsin Medical School, to ask me to develop a mini-fellowship program, entitled "Advanced Obstetrics," which would be offered to physicians from the United States and Canada who were already in practice but felt the need for upgrading their obstetric skills. Again, my Green Bay colleagues and I agreed, and the mini-fellowships began in 1985. The fellows were integrated into the residents' call schedules and also participated in the daily morning meetings.

In 2000, when Aurora constructed the fourth Green Bay hospital (which we didn't need) we lost some of our good teachers and their patients from the resident and mini-fellowship teaching programs. To avoid short-changing family medicine residents enrolled in our Advanced Obstetrics Rotation, we had to discontinue our mini-fellowship program that year. From 1985 to its final year in 2000, approximately 170 physicians in practice participated in this two-week mini-fellowship program.

University of Wisconsin Medical School's Continuing Medical Education (CME) Chairman Tom Meyer nicely summarized the 15-year history of our mini-fellowship program in his letter supporting me for the WMAA RALPH HAWLEY DISTINGUISHED SERVICE AWARD:

The University of Wisconsin Madison

September 1, 2004
Karen S. Peterson, Executive Director
Medical Alumni Association
Re: Herbert F. Sandmire, MD
Dear Ms. Peterson:

I would like to add my strongest support to the nomination of Dr. Sandmire for the RALPH HAWLEY DISTINGUISHED SERVICE AWARD.

Dr. Sandmire has long been a strong supporter of the UW Medical School in general and the Office of Continuing Medical Education (CME) in particular. During the 30 years that I directed that Office, I turned to Dr. Sandmire on many occasions for assistance in both teaching and solving problems which arose related to our activities.

Perhaps the most significant contribution Dr. Sandmire made to the UW CME Program was between 1985 and 2000. Dr. Sandmire and his group allowed us to offer a rigorous two week "Visiting Fellowship" in Normal Obstetrics for practicing physicians. This was a tightly constructed curriculum which ensured that the registrants covered the essential didactic material and, most important, actually delivered up to 12 babies under close supervision during the two-week Visiting Fellowship. It is my belief that this was the only location in the USA that such an opportunity was available to US physicians who wished to return to OB practice or whose hospitals had concern about their ability to deal with normal obstetric problems. Alas, the program ended in 2000 because of an insufficient number of patients to support the Green Bay OB Residency rotation and the Visiting Fellowships. The Office of CME still gets requests for the program which we are unable to fulfill. I believe that if the CME Office were granted one Visiting Fellowship, we would choose the program in Normal Obstetrics as the one which would serve the greatest demand for practicing physicians.

I have long wished to be able to do more than say "thanks" to Dr. Sandmire for arranging and administering that program and believe this would acknowledge his contributions – hence my strong support for his candidacy for the Ralph Hawley award.

Yours sincerely,
Thomas C. Meyer, MD
Prof. Emeritus, Dept of Pediatrics and Continuing Medical Education

The following excerpts from the winter/spring 1989 issue of *Perinatal Pages* describes the experience of one of our visiting Fellows:

OB Fellowship: A Personal Reflection by Tom Wex, MD

Editors' Note: As a follow-up to the article "Visiting Fellowship in Obstetrics," by Dr. Herbert Sandmire one of the OB fellows has given us a brief account of his experience in the program. Dr. Tom Wex, a family practicianer, participated in the program during August 1988:

The OB fellow is in an unusual position because he only has two weeks to accomplish his goals. Those goals may very well differ from fellow to fellow, but I think they will always include a desire for hands-on experience. To get that experience, a resident has a longer time than a fellow to establish himself with the attending physicians. However, I was pleasantly surprised to find the opportunity to participate in many procedures while at St. Vincent and Bellin hospitals. I was able to perform 14 deliveries, observe another 11 and assist with 7 C-sections. That reflects not only a very busy OB service, but also a lot of trust from the attending physician.

In addition to the clinical experiences available, there was also an opportunity to refresh my "book" knowledge of obstetrics. Reading materials were provided and morning conferences were held with Dr. Sandmire.

Back in Madison, I feel the fellowship will enhance the OB portion of my family practice. I'd like to thank everyone for making my two weeks so worthwhile.

Appleton Family Practice
225 S. Morrison St.
Appleton, WI 54911-5760

November 16, 1992
Mr. Joseph Neidenbach
St. Vincent Hospital
Dear Neidenbach,
I just recently completed an OB Fellowship with Dr. Sandmire at Bellin and St. Vincent's. Educationally this has been one of the most beneficial things I have been able to do in continuing medical education in a long time.

I want to commend your staff on the labor and delivery floor, the nursery, and the post partum unit for their willingness to be involved

*in the teaching process, their cheerful care of patients, and their effi-
ciency in carrying out their activities.*

*I further would like to thank the hospital for sponsoring the lodg-
ing at the Coachlight Inn. I wasn't able to be there very often because
of my labor duties but it was always there and was a nice place to
"crash." I appreciated also the access to the physician lounge and meals
when they were provided.*

*I applaud your hospital for its participation in this worthwhile
educational activity. I would have no hesitation to recommend it
highly to anyone interested in upgrading their OB skills.*

Sincerely, John N. Allhiser, M.D., Associate Director

CHAPTER 25

Remedial work

STARTING IN 1985, our mini-fellowship program broadened its sphere to train physicians in practice who were judged by the Wisconsin Medical Examining Board (MEB) to need remedial work. As such, Dr. Meyer, working on behalf of the State Board, began sending physicians in need of remedial work our way. So it happened that our residency program led to the mini-fellowship program, which, in turn, led to my devising and carrying out remedial programs for the MEB.

In 1985, I realized I was overloaded with teaching responsibilities, particularly the time required to write supporting statements for students or physicians who had come to Green Bay to participate in one of the three programs for which I was responsible. After 20 years and 250 students, I relinquished the preceptorship work in 1985. As a result of my long tenure as volunteer "preceptor in charge," I received the Max Fox Preceptor Award that year. The inscription on the back of the chair read, "for your dedicated and effective service to University of Wisconsin medical students as a preceptor in charge. (1966-1985)"

During that same time I also received the 1985 Erwin R. Schmidt Interstate Teaching Award, sponsored by the Interstate Postgraduate Medical Association of North America. This award is presented to "a Wisconsin physician who has distinguished himself in the teaching of medical students and physicians in practice."

The mechanism by which the MEB determined the physicians in need for remedial work was interesting. I recall Dr. Wooley, who had some issues with the Minnesota MEB on the basis of a physician-nurse conflict and who absolutely did not need any remedial program. Nevertheless, he carried out his required assignment, and during the time he was with me, we co-authored and published a paper entitled

"Macrosomia: Can We Prevent Big Problems With Big Babies?" Other out-of-state physicians in need of remedial work came from Michigan.

I was given wide latitude in the development of the remedial program, testing it to determine its effectiveness and making a final determination if the physician would continue to be licensed in Wisconsin – as can be seen by the excerpts below regarding training stipulations set forth by the Wisconsin MEB in the case of respondent Dr. Mustansir Majeed:

> *Respondent shall retain Dr. Herbert F. Sandmire to test Respondent on a minimum of six obstetrical case scenarios following completion of the education required by paragraph 2.a. of this Order. The testing shall include the reading and interpretation of fetal monitor strips, and explanation by Respondent of how Respondent would manage each situation. Dr. Sandmire shall prepare a written report on the testing and recommendations for Respondent's training in light of these results, which report shall be delivered to the Department Monitor for review by a member of the Board. If Dr. Sandmire recommends that Respondent should pursue additional training to achieve minimal competence in obstetrics, Respondent shall complete that training without further order of the Board, and Respondent shall repeat the requirements of this paragraph of this Order, but limited to retesting of the topic or topics Dr. Sandmire previously recommended. When Dr. Sandmire reports to the Department Monitor that Respondent has demonstrated minimal competence on the testing Dr. Sandmire administers, the Respondent will have met the Board's requirements and his license will have no restrictions.*

The following correspondence from Dr. Majeed's attorney, Ms. Ratzel, indicates closure for MEB v. Majeed, M.D.:

> *Dear Dr. Sandmire,*
> *Dr. Majeed completed the additional CME course work and has completed all elements of the Stipulation with the MEB – there are no restrictions on his license.*
> *Thank you again for all of your help. You are a wonderful mentor. There are few – actually there are no other physicians willing to give so much of their time to help fellow physicians. I wish I could nominate you for a very special award.*
> *You may discard all of the materials.*
> *Many thanks, again, and very Best Wishes.*
> *Mary Lee Ratzel*

Other physicians who I have helped are identified in the following letters:

vmondloch@wi.rr.com

4/21/2005
Dr. Sandmire,
I received verbal notification from my attorney that the Medical Examining Board has agreed to accept the clarification that was forwarded to them regarding my educational program and that they will be lifting the educational restriction on my medical license.

I want to thank you wholeheartedly for your time and efforts expended on my behalf. Without your help, I'm certain that I would not have been in a position to challenge and work toward this hurdle. The state truly needs to have such a group of dedicated physicians who are in a position to help and are able to take the time from their own practice to offer such help. Thank you again,
Vicki Mondloch MD

John Waeltz MD
4773 N. Cramer St.
Milwaukee, WI 53211

November 18, 2006
Dear Dr. Sandmire,
I wish to sincerely thank you for all that you have done for me. The afternoon spent in study and review was a very memorable time. Your advocacy was critical to finally clearing my license from the "catch 22"" to recertify and document my competency to the licensing board. Your expertise and unselfish sharing of your time is so appreciated. Attorney Mary Lee Ratzel has revealed that you did not desire compensation. You have my deep respect and admiration. I am in your debt. The afternoon was exciting for me on a professional level for the depth of the review of obstetrics. It was also special on a personal level to see a fellow physician exemplify his devotion to teaching and patient care.

I have enjoyed your articles and wished to compliment you on their conclusions.

Again, thank you for your time, advocacy and support.
Sincerely, John Woeltz

Another example of my helping an obstetrician from out of Wisconsin is the following letter from Brian J.Bell MD from Michigan:

Brian J. Bell, MD, FACOG
401 North Shore Drive
South Haven, MI 49090
January 15, 2002

Dear Dr. Sandmire:
I received notification from Brian Stephenson of Garan, Lucow, Miller, P.C. that you have elected not to bill for your work on my behalf in the Alpena General Hospital case. I want to express my sincere gratitude for this most magnanimous gesture. As you are aware I have been paying the legal expenses out of pocket and your selfless act helps tremendously in this time of financial hardship.
Once again I can't thank you enough for your generosity. May God bless you.
Sincerely,
Brian J. Bell, MD

Paul Haupt was another physician who benefitted from our remedial teaching program:

Menominee Medical Clinic
Paul Haupt D.O., Harold Grissinger M.D,. William Hultman, PA-C
1100 Tenth St.
Menominee, Michigan 49858
August 21, 1996
Dear Drs. Sandmire and DeMott,
I am writing to let you know how much I appreciated your help in achieving my goal of having the obstetrics restriction lifted from my license. On Monday, 08/19/96, I received an Order from the Wisconsin Medical Board reversing the restriction on my license, based on a letter they received from Dr. Meyer, Director of CME at University of Wisconsin, Madison, and I also wanted to let you know how much I appreciated your help.
The program you have established in obstetrics in Green Bay is one of the finest educational experiences I have had in my career. Certainly, the volume of obstetrics and the quality of supervision is second to none. The program is set up in a very professional manner, and the academic aspect is clearly equal to the clinical experience in my opinion. Also, the nursing staff of both hospitals was extremely helpful in

169

aiding the educational process and I thought that you should know this. It is quite clear that in spite of your busy clinical schedules, you have devoted a significant portion of your energies and dedication to education. I would also like you to express my thanks to Drs. Bechtel and Cavanaugh as well as many of the other staff obstetricians who allowed me to participate in the care of their patients.

It is very reassuring for me to know that there are physicians such as yourselves as willing to help a colleague in the mid-portion of his career as they are to help their patients on a day-to-day basis. This experience has not only improved my obstetrical skills I believe, but also has restored quite a bit of my enthusiasm for the practice of medicine. Please be aware that I am deeply grateful for your help in this situation and that I have been making others aware of the quality educational program that you have established in Green Bay.

My best wishes to you in all future endeavors,
Paul A. Haupt, D.O.

I am honored and humbled by the MEB's recognition of my teaching ability and their request for me to develop remedial programs for colleagues in need. Incidentally, over the past 25 years, I have never charged a colleague for my time - even those from other states. As I mentioned earlier, I believe that the activities we engage in without remuneration can be the most rewarding.

In some cases, I was asked by a physician's attorney to review the MEB's complaint to see if the physician's care was indeed beneath expected standards. If I found the care was acceptable, I would testify before the Department of Regulations and Licensing on behalf of the physician, as I did in the case of the Wisconsin MEB v. Dr. Jacqueline Irland, presided over by administrative law Judge Jeffrey D. Boldt. A Ms. Rude had filed a complaint with the MEB against Irland, a Milwaukee obstetrician, alleging that there was a delay in the diagnosis of breast cancer that developed during the time she was nursing her baby. During lactation it is exceedingly difficult to distinguish cancerous lumps from normal breast tissue that is engorged with milk.

Madison physician Susan Davidson and I testified on behalf of Dr. Irland, while Dr. Klaus Diem, also from Madison, testified that Dr. Irland's care fell below the minimal standards. Judge Boldt's ruling was based upon several "findings of fact," some of which are listed below:

Whatever Ms. Rude felt in her breast in March 2003, it could not have been the cancer that was diagnosed in November 2003. (Sandmire at 1073-1075)

It is very common for professors to use the ACOG Guidelines in teaching residents. (Sandmire at 1109)

Ms. Rude's tumor could not have been palpable in May, 2003 under any circumstances. (Sandmire at 1073-1075, 1138)

Using a 65-day doubling time calculation, Ms. Rude's tumor would have been 0.25 cm in May. (Sandmire at 1073)

Using the more conservative 130-day calculation, Ms. Rude's cancer would have been 0.5 cm in May. (Sandmire at 1073-1075)

At her deposition, testifying under oath, Ms. Rude denied telling Dr. Walker that she initially noted a problem in her breast in July or August 2003. (Rude Dep., Ex. 238 at 104)

Exhibit 244 shows that is exactly what Ms. Rude told Dr. Walker in December 2003. (Ex. 244; Rude at 212)

Judge Boldt's "Discussion" read as follows:

On the standard of care and other issues, the Respondent (accused physician) presented the testimony of Dr. Herbert Sandmire and Dr. Susan Davidson—two very distinguished practicing OB/GYN's. Dr. Sandmire is a widely published and respected obstetrician with over five decades of experience. The Medical Examining Board has authorized Dr. Sandmire to implement remedial education programs for physicians who need them. He serves as a reviewer for seven different medical journals, including the "American Journal of Obstetrics & Gynecology and The New England Journal of Medicine." (Sandmire at 1018-19). Dr. Sandmire very recently won the American College of Obstetrics and Gynecologists ("ACOG's") Lifetime Distinguished Service Award. (Sandmire at 1025; Exs. 235, 235A). Dr. Davidson is renowned for her resident teaching activities, and has won the University of Wisconsin's Clinical Teacher of the Year Award three times. Davidson has been authorized by the Department of Regulation and Licensing to review patient complaints and determine whether prosecutions should go forward. (Davidson at 893-894; Ex. 236)

The ACOG Guidelines represent the consensus of ACOG's broad and diverse membership at the point in time at which the Guidelines are published. The Guidelines are updated as the practice of medicine evolves. (Sandmire at 1172-1173)

The trier of fact (Judge Boldt) agrees with Dr. Irland that "compliance with ACOG's standards per se satisfies the "minimal standards" test applicable in this proceeding. The Testimony of Respondent's experts that Dr. Irland complied fully with the 2003 ACOG Guidelines was unimpeachable and largely uncontroverted. (Sandmire at 1050; Davidson at 919-21 0)

This brings us to the second major weakness in the state's case, namely the testimony of Dr. Sandmire which raised strong doubts on the inference of the Division that the lump felt by Dr. Irland in May was the same one that was later diagnosed as cancer.

As Dr. Sandmire testified, civil courts have long used the "scientific probabilities" expressed in expected "doubling times" as the best evidence of the size of cancers at particular intervals in time. (Sandmire at 1071) Dr. Sandmire opined categorically that Dr. Irland "wasn't feeling cancer (in May, 2003). She was feeling fibrocystic changes." (Sandmire at 1136) The reason for this strong opinion was Dr. Sandmire's judgment that Ms. Rude's tumor could not have been of sufficient size to be palpable in May 2003 under any circumstances. (Sandmire at 107301075, 1138)

Using a 65-day doubling time calculation, Ms. Rude's tumor would have been 0.25 cm in May. (Sandmire at 1073) Using the more conservative 130-day calculation, Ms. Rude's cancer would have been 0.5 cm in May. (Sandmire at 1073-1075) A 0.5 cm breast tumor cannot be perceived by palpation and 1 centimeter is the generally-accepted threshold at which a breast cancer can begin to be observed by palpation. (Diem at 649; Sandmire at 1074-1075; Walker at 522-523)

Ms. Rude likewise believes that she is doing an important service in raising awareness about the diagnosis of breast cancer in pregnant women. However, sincerity of purpose and a laudable public health goal cannot be had at the expense of fairness to Dr. Irland. While we understand the reasons which motivated this prosecution, the Division of Enforcement has not carried its burden of proof in this matter.

It would be fundamentally unfair and against the greater weight of the evidence to discipline Dr. Irland under these circumstances.

In the end, the judge noted in his "Conclusions of Law" that the "Respondent has not committed unprofessional conduct as defined by Wis. Admin. Code & MED 10.02(2)(h) and is not subject to discipline under Wis. Stat. & 448.02(3)."

While it was certainly good that an individual patient with a grievance was able to be heard and have her "day in court," Ms. Rude's untruthful testimony in her deposition did not help her cause, and through the misguided efforts of Klaus Diem and Sandra Nowack, Attorney for the Department of Regulation and Licensing, the process was allowed to go on too long at great expense and time invested. Furthermore, this investigation of questionable merit, lasting over a few years, was emotionally draining for the accused physician.

CHAPTER 26

Spangenberg / Gerhard baby

I HAD FINISHED my internship at William Beaumont Hospital on July 1, 1954 and was assigned to the Obstetric Department at Ladd Air Force Base Hospital, Fairbanks, Alaska the next month. Since I had had no post-internship training in any specialty, I was categorized as a general medical officer. With the end of the Korean War, many specialists were completing their tour of duty and replaced by general medical officers like me. This provided me with six months of excellent, intensive, supervised training by those three residency-trained obstetricians, prior to their rotating home. I benefited from the tutoring I received regarding the indications for and correct use of forceps as well as how to perform a cesarean section. At the end of that intense, six-month training period, at age 25, I was appointed Chief of the Obstetric Department.

On September 30, 1954, under the excellent assistance and supervision of Dr. Winterhalter, I performed my first cesarean birth on Jean Spangenberg, wife of an army sergeant. Dr. Winterhalter was very patient with me, telling me where and how to place each stitch in closing the uterine and abdominal wall incisions. In appreciation of his help, I pledged myself to be equally patient when in the future I would be assisting a younger, less experienced doctor in the performance of a cesarean or any other operation. Over the ensuing 30 years, I had many opportunities to assist younger doctors with their performance of cesarean births, and to help them relax I would recount my first cesarean birth experience and the amount of assistance I needed, always mentioning the patient's name was Spangenberg.

Much later in Green Bay, during the latter part her pregnancy, Kathy Gerhard, in 1984, reading her baby book which detailed all the vital happenings in her early life, she found that a Dr. Herbert F. Sandmire was listed as the attending physician at her birth. Having just come across this information, she was seeing my partner, Dr. Cavanaugh, for a routine prenatal visit and asked him if the Herbert F. Sandmire in her baby book could be the same doctor as the one who is your partner in this office. I remember distinctly Dr. Cavanaugh calling up the hallway, "Herb, did you do a cesarean on a woman in Alaska in 1954?" I responded, "Was her name Spangenberg?" whereupon he asked Kathy Gerhard her maiden name and, lo and behold, she said, "Spangenberg." Cavanaugh then responded saying, "Yes." He at that time thought I had a remarkable memory to remember Kathy's mother's name, having not seen her for 30 years. Later I told him that she was my first cesarean birth and the rest of the story.

Kathy was Dr. Cavanaugh's patient, but coincidentally, I was on call when she went into labor, and I had the good fortune of attending the birth of her child at 9:05 AM Sunday, September 30, 1984 – on Kathy's 30th birthday - three decades after I performed the cesarean for her own birth. I later found out that Kathy was Crystal's dental hygienist.

The *Green Bay Press Gazette* had a front-page report entitled, "Small World, Sandmire first delivered Mom, now her baby," along with a beautiful color photograph. Kathy's parents, residing in Milwaukee, came up for the delivery, and we renewed our acquaintance. The *Green Bay Press Gazette* further reported that the "Sunday birth wasn't the only one that brought back memories for Sandmire. Last Friday he attended the delivery of a second generation when a son was born to Lisa and J. Antonio Gonzales, 2651 He-Nis-Ra-Lane. . . . He also had delivered Mrs. Gonzales, the daughter of Lew and Ann Carpenter, on May 12, 1962, in Green Bay."

Green Bay Packer fans will remember Lew Carpenter as a Packer running back during the Green Bay Packer Glory Years which were chronicled earlier in this manuscript. We were saddened by an article in the *Green Bay Press Gazette* November 15, 2010 reporting that Lew Carpenter had passed away at age 78.

Eight days after the *Green Bay Press Gazette* "Small World" article, there was a letter to the editor with the headline, "Criticizes doctor story." This was a common tactic for those who do not believe in women's reproductive rights. The letter read:

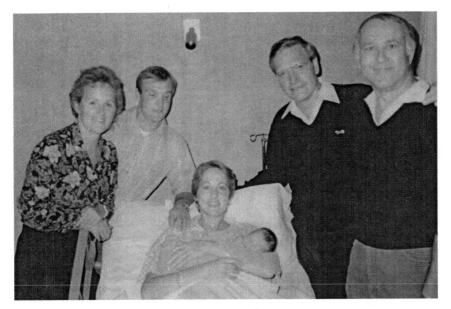

Kathy's parents, Richard and Jean Spangenberg came to Green Bay from Milwaukee to celebrate the birth of their grandchild. (September 30, 1984)

I'm writing a comment to the story in the Press-Gazette, October 2, concerning Dr. Herbert Sandmire delivering a baby.

Considering that he and/or his associates are the only abortion doctors in Green Bay, this story is a mockery to the human race.

The article made him look and sound like an admirable human being. Have we so little regard for our fellow human beings that we admire a man who does what he does for money!

I feel sorrow and shame for all of us. How far advanced our intellectualism has gotten us that we dispose of unwanted and imperfect human beings and then applaud the people who carry out this heinous act. Darlene Williams, 1155 Sharie Lane.

CHAPTER 27

$\mathcal{P}$articipation in medical and other organizations

High school reunions

I commuted to Madison East High School from Cottage Grove and graduated in 1946, the year after World War II ended. I attended all of my high school reunions with the exception of the 1956 reunion, during which time I was in Iowa City in my residency. Also, I did not go when, in 2006, they started having them at noon as if we were "old folks"!!

Wisconsin Medical Alumni Association (WMAA)

Following my graduation from the University of Wisconsin School of Medicine in 1953, I became a life member of WMAA and participated actively in that organization, serving on the board of directors from 1985 to 1993 and as president in 1989 and 1990. In 1985 I received the WMAA "Max Fox Preceptorship Award," "for [my] dedicated and effective service to University of Wisconsin medical students as a preceptor in charge" (1966-1985). In 2005, the WMAA presented me with the "Ralph Hawley Distinguished Service Award," recognizing my "contributions to [my] community, to [my] profession and to a broad segment of society." Another Medical Alumni Association that I was a member of was the Iowa OB/Gyn Alumni Association, serving as President in 1978.

As part of my responsibilities as President of the WMAA beginning in the spring of 1989, I authored six articles for the *Alumni Quarterly* entitled "Now I know," "What am I doing here?" "Ask Ralph," "A man called Jacob," "President's column," and "I'm still listening."

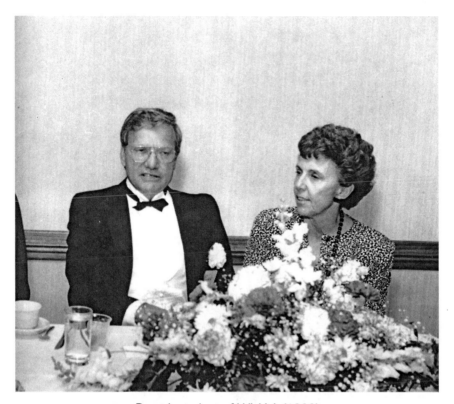

President-elect of WMAA (1988)

The "What am I doing here?" article best captures my thoughts at that time:

President's Column
What am I doing here?

Approximately two years ago I attended a movie with Crystal and two grown – not living at home – children and a daughter-in-law. While waiting about 15 minutes for the feature to start, I experienced an acute awareness of having made a mistake in going and exclaimed, "What am I doing here?" The family broke out in laughter – not derisive but not sympathetic – perhaps suspenseful. All being amateur

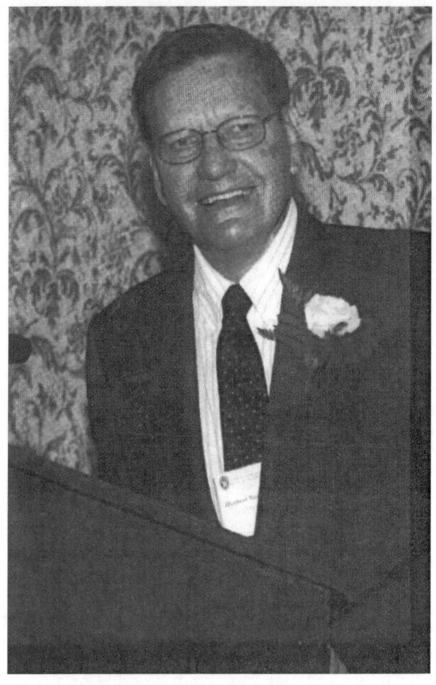

Receiving the WMAA 2005 Ralph Hawley Distinguished Service Award.

scientists especially in the soft disciplines, they had an opportunity to observe developing anxiety in an unabashed, fully admitted, compulsive workaholic.

Time management for busy professionals becomes increasingly important. Our younger colleagues have both spousal and parenting responsibilities and we older physicians continue to have spousal responsibilities. Mostly, professional obligations have won the battle against the family in the contest for the busy physician's time. Wives or husbands have survived this through adjustment, adaptation or resignation leading to at least partial acceptance in not all but most cases. How we allocate the hours available should depend on the proportionate satisfaction experienced as a result of our various activities.

Currently we are often compelled to engage in non-productive and unpleasant experiences – like explaining to an insurance company nurse in some distant city, why I am not going to do a pre-hysterectomy biopsy on a patient with a D&C diagnosis (mega-biopsy) of atypical adenomatous endometrial hyperplasia. Government regulations often produce frustrating distractions which interfere with patient care. Medical legal risks result in endless defensive medical tactics, all of which are time consuming and increase costs without care enhancement. Some preoperative and other patient care notes sound more like a brief prepared for the United States Supreme Court than a description of a patient's condition and recommendations for its management.

How do physicians cope with all of the negatives of modern medical practice? Obviously we need to develop and enhance offsetting positive satisfying experiences. My prescription for a response to all those "bastards" who want to do us in is to take refuge in time-proven, satisfying, professional activities:

1. *Make an obsession of delivering the best, most caring cost effective care possible. (Battle our adversaries through kindness and competence using Patients as our warriors.)*
2. *Allocate time to sharing your knowledge and experience with others. Some people call this teaching. Regardless of your definition, it is a true, time-honored, self-satisfying activity.*
3. *Record and tabulate some of your clinical observations and present and publish your findings – research.*
4. *Assiduously maintain and improve our profession by helping attract young people to our medical schools.*

Not surprisingly, Numbers 2 and 3 above, substantially increase the possibility of achieving Number 1. Number 4 represents the main current focus of our alumni association through the development of a low and deferred interest student loan fund. Also needed is for physicians in practice to share their positive experiences with talented young people in their community.

So, what am I doing here – writing this column?: Engaging in a self-satisfying experience...

The movie alluded to in the above column was "Peggy Sue Got Married." Prior to that, the most recent movie I had seen was "Chariots of Fire" in 1982 while visiting my father in Tampa, Florida. After "Peggy Sue Got Married," I didn't hit the theater again until 2010, when we saw Green Bay native Tony Shaloub's "Feed the Fish." *According to this schedule my next movie attendance will be in 2018.*

Booklet for 45th Med Sch reunion

The following current activities of Herb Sandmire can be found in the booklet prepared for the Medical School class of 1953 just prior to our 45th reunion in May, 1998.

Herb Sandmire

Another non-retiree, he continues practicing gynecology, teaching, and serving as an expert witness. He really enjoys tangling with those lawyers and Crys is always on hand for moral support. Crys is CEO of Crystal Condo Properties, a partnership with their five children and eight grandchildren who are scattered from Oregon to Maine. Herb's most memorable med school experience was dating some girls and the most forgettable was dating some other girls. His advice is:

I. *Be cordial – live longer.*

II. *Be happy.*

III. *Live in harmony with your environment (he rides a bike to his office).*

IV. *Lose weight .*

V. *Laughter is contagious, catch it.*

VI. *Limit sex to once daily.*

VII. *Avoid the following IQ deductions:*

    A. *wearing a baseball cap: 5*

    B. *drinking bottled water: 5*

    C. *smoking: 20*

    D. *patronizing casinos: 10*

    E. *owning a gas guzzling automobile : 20*

F.   *believing vaccinations are a hoax: 10*
G.   *patronizing "health food" stores: 10*
      Maximum total deductions: 80

Herbert and Crystal Sandmire plaque

At the Middleton Society dinner on October 22, 2004, a plaque with a picture of Sweetie and me was unveiled as part of the Middleton Society Wall of Honor in Alumni Hall. The inscription below our picture was:

> *We both have had the good fortune to receive our higher education through the University of Wisconsin. In appreciation for the quality of that experience we have welcomed the opportunity of giving something back. Dr. Sandmire also appreciates his opportunities to participate in the education of medical students as a Preceptor and of residents as Director of the Green Bay Obstetric rotation.*
> *Crystal J. Sandmire B.A., UWGB 1980*
> *Herbert F. Sandmire B.S., UW 1950; M.D. 1953*

The plaque was in appreciation for our donations through membership in the Middleton and Bardeen Societies together with numerous other random donations.

Rhine cruise on the Rembrandt, June 9-19, 2006

The University of Wisconsin Medical School and the Wisconsin Medical Alumni (WMAA) sponsored a celebration Rhine cruise in June of 2006. The historic events celebrated included the 100th year of the medical school and the 50th year for WMAA. Invitations were sent to members of the UW Medical School faculty and the WMAA. Sweetie and I, along with four of our five children (Cheryl, Yvonne, Mike and Dave), joined 63 others on this once-in-a-lifetime celebration cruise.

Medical School Dean Farrell and other faculty members provided occasional lectures during the cruise. Dean Farrell gave his "state of the medical school" address, describing all of the changes that occurred during his tenure.

Our cruise began at Basel, Switzerland and ended ten days later at Amsterdam. On day three, we arrived at Breisach, Germany where we were provided with a full day bus tour of the Black Forest. Late that afternoon we arrived in Strasbourg, France. Most of our meals were on board and were wonderful. The next day we toured Strasbourg.

Sweetie and I were acquainted with several of our co-passengers who seemed to enjoy the opportunity to see two generations of our family. The six of us always "hanging out" together made quite an impression on our cruise mates. Someone, probably Professor Patrick McBride (same age as our kids) started greeting us by saying "All Sandmires, all of the time." Mike and Dave positively enjoyed fooling-around with Patrick, mimicking German pronouncements and enunciations from a prior serial television show. Years prior, during the mid-1980s, Dr. McBride had enrolled in a mini-fellowship in obstetrics under my direction in Green Bay.

On the fifth day, we departed from Strasbourg, cruising down the Rhine to Greffen for a city tour. That afternoon we arrived at Speyer, Germany.

The highlight of our cruise occurred on Day six, Wednesday, June 14 with our arrival at Heidelberg for a full-day tour of the city, including its famous castle.

The remainder of the cruise was filled with beautiful scenery, including numerous castles on each side of the river and stops in Mainz, Koblenz, Cologne, Arnhem and Amsterdam. We appreciated seeing so much with only one unpacking and one packing up for the entire 10 days.

In Amsterdam, our friends, the Lammertsma family from Zaandam, Holland, came to our ship, the Rembrandt, accompanied us on a canal trip, and had lunch with us at a restaurant on the river. It was great to renew our friendship with them (see the Chapter, Foreign Friends where I have more information about this family).

We were sad to have our wonderful, enjoyable cruise come to an end. Even though we tried to pretend otherwise, the farewell reception and dinner on the Rembrandt brought us back to reality.

Brown County Medical Society

I attended most of the meetings and served as delegate to the annual meeting of the Wisconsin State Medical Society for many years.

Closer to home, our Brown County Medical Society was a smaller organization – so small that in 1964, Crystal and I, along with the Meyers and Harts, co-hosted a buffet supper, at our house ,for its 80 members and their spouses.

Wisconsin State Medical Society (WI SMS)

In 1969, I received an award for my poster presentation (*Intrauterine contraceptive device*) at the State Medical Society's annual meeting. In 1985, I received the "Irwin R. Schmidt Interstate Teaching Award," sponsored by the Interstate Postgraduate Medical Association of North America. This award is presented to a physician who has distinguished himself in teaching medical students and physicians in practice. In 1993, the WI-SMS presented me with its "Wisconsin Service Recognition Award."

I have, since 1968, served on WI-SMS study committee on maternal mortality. In addition, I served as chairman of the commission on public information from 1977 to 1982 and as a member of the commission on medical liability from 1987 to 1993.

Eight of my 47 peer-reviewed articles have been published in the *Wisconsin State Medical Journal.*

I was nominated for the office of President-Elect of the WI-SMS in 1981. As a candidate, I drafted the following areas of concern that I believed should be addressed by the State Medical Society.

1. *Another emerging crisis due to a proliferation of malpractice actions. If this continues, we will soon reach the time when any but perfect results will automatically result in malpractice action. In my view, major legislative action is needed.*

2. *We need to be much more effective in providing cost effective medical care.*

3. *We need better "public relations" techniques in most of our Wisconsin physicians' offices.*

4. *We need to continue to work toward better physician distribution.*

5. *We need more active involvement by younger physicians in State Medical Society activities.*

6. *We need to continue the improvement in our working relationships with media persons.*

7. *We need to continue to explore relationships with representatives of business, industry, and labor directed toward a cooperative effort in solving health care delivery and cost problems.*

The following letter from Dr. Griffin of Mauston is an example of physicians supporting my candidacy.

Vernon M. Griffin M.D., S.C.
Corporate Business Office
767 Elm Street
March 30, 1981
Herbert F. Sandmire M.D.
704 S. Webster Ave.
Green Bay, WI 54301
Dear Friend Herb,
Everyone here is most pleased that you will run for the office of President Elect of the SMS. As you learned when Dr. Lewis spoke with you and Dr. Riesch, the office is supposed to be for a doctor outside district 1 (Milwaukee) this coming time. Therefore let me join with others in again urging you to run this time.
Hope you like my bum typing.
Yours, Griff

The Milwaukee members,of the nominating, having a seven-to-six majority, determined that it would not "look good" to have pickets surrounding the office of the WI-SMS president - this despite the fact that the Society's House of Delegates reaffirmed a woman's right to have an abortion the previous year. The Milwaukee physicians' selection of one of their own was in violation of the unwritten agreement that a Milwaukee physician would be nominated only every three years. Former SMS President Russell Lewis, confided in me his concerns about this in the following letter:

Department of Obstetrics and Gynecology, Marshfield Clinic
April 5, 1982
Dear Herb,
I thought I'd put this in a separate letter, but as long as I was writing to you anyway I thought I should report to you a rather disturbing conversation that took place at Madison at a recent meeting involving physicians in the State Medical Society. It came up because there was a question raised about Dr. Ervin coming up to Milwaukee's turn to have the presidency, and specifically the question was raised as to what had hurt you and your candidacy. The answer was the abortion issue. I had never given that any serious thought, but the feeling that was expressed there was that as long as you were doing abortions, and as long as people were marching outside of your Surgi-

Center on occasion, that the State Medical Society would be in a potentially embarrassing position, should you become the President. At least several people in attendance at this meeting, who obviously have to remain anonymous, stated that they did not see how the Society could, under these circumstances, propose you for the office of President-Elect.

Since this was sort of a new and startling situation to me, and because you might consider further activity along this line, I thought that as an old friend who had been somewhat involved in the previous candidacy I thought that you should know this attitude existed, and may well have a bearing on any future thought and activities you might have.

Sincerely yours, Russell F. Lewis MD

The American Medical Association (AMA)

Except for having one of my papers published in the *Journal of the American Medical Association*, I did not participate in its activities.

Wisconsin Society of Obstetrics and Gynecology, later to become the Wisconsin section of American Congress of Obstetricians and Gynecologists (WI-ACOG)

This was my favorite organization and the one receiving more of my participation than any other. The first meeting I attended was in 1959, and since then I have attended every one of the ensuing 50 meetings. At approximately one-third of those meetings, I presented a paper.

I served as chairman of the Professional Relations and Liability Committee from 1983 to 2008. Part of my responsibilities included (from 1986 to 2008) getting a summary of all OB-Gyn suits filed in Wisconsin and categorizing them according to the alleged negligence. A summary of my annual reports was presented to the WI-ACOG annual meeting and was also included in the organization's newsletter.

On July 21, 1988, I teamed up with Peter Hickey, a very good defense attorney, in presenting a pre-convention workshop entitled "The role and responsibility of the expert witness in OB-Gyn claims." I served as President of the organization in 1972.

ACOG awards

A copy of the following press release, written by Robert Jaeger M.D., Chairman of Wisconsin Section ACOG, was mailed to me in early July, 1995. I was honored to be the first recipient of the newly established WI-ACOG Distinguished Service Award.

The American College of Obstetricians and Gynecologists, District VI
Office of the Chairman of the Wisconsin Section

July 1995
Green Bay Press Gazette
Green Bay, Wisconsin 54307-9430
Subject: Press Release
Dear Sirs:
At the combined annual meeting of the Wisconsin Society of Obstetrics and Gynecology, and the Wisconsin Section of the American College of Obstetrics and Gynecology, Dr. Herbert F. Sandmire of Green Bay was awarded the <u>Society's Distinguished Service Award</u>. The text of the presentation follows:

"The Advisory Council has established the <u>Distinguished Service Award</u> to honor members of the society for meritorious service in the advancement of medical science, medical education, and medical care, and in recognition of service to the physicians of the section and the people of Wisconsin. This highest award of the section is not to be presented annually, but only when the Advisory Council approves a candidate nominated by the fellows of the section."

"It is most fitting that the first recipient of the award is Dr. Herbert F. Sandmire. As you know, Herb has made numerous contributions of original research to the medical literature, and is an active teacher of nurses, a preceptor to medical students, and a mentor to resident physicians. He has served as a president of this society and of the University of Wisconsin Medical Alumni Association, and as an officer in numerous professional organizations. This award recognizes all these contributions, but especially Herb's efforts toward medical-legal fair treatment for the physicians of Wisconsin. Whether assisting individual physicians at the most trying hour of their professional lives, educating colleagues in risk management, lobbying the state assembly, senate and governor, or pressing the state medical society to promote effective, appropriate and reasonable tort reform, his dedication, persistence, and indomitable good humor are in no small measure responsible for the tort reforms recently signed by Governor Thompson. It is with admiration and gratitude the Advisory Council presents the Distinguished Service Award to Dr. Herbert F. Sandmire."

Dr. Sandmire received the award with his usual self effacing humor. Commenting "my wife will ask if there has been some mistake."

Sincerely,
Robert Jaeger, Chairman of the WI Section of ACOG

On May 20, 2008, I received the following letter from the Executive Secretary of Wisconsin Section of ACOG informing me that I had again been chosen to receive the Distinguished Service Award:

Wisconsin Section, American College of Obstetricians & Gynecologists
P.O. Box 636, Pewaukee WI 53072-0636

May 20, 2008
Dear Dr. Sandmire,
It is with great pleasure that I inform you that you have again been chosen to receive a Distinguished Service Award for your many years of dedicated service to the Wisconsin Section/ACOG.
The Advisory Council would like to present this award to you at the Annual Business Meeting on Saturday, July 19th, 2008 at the Kalahari Resort in Wisconsin Dells.
Your tireless efforts in compiling and presenting facts that help the practicing physician maintain the quality of the specialty of obstetrics and gynecology is appreciated by all.
As our guest your registration fees will be waived.
I look forward to seeing you and Mrs. Sandmire at the 2008 annual meeting.
Sincerely, Dawn M. Maerker, Executive Secretary

The American College of Obstetricians and Gynecology (ACOG) Distinguished Service Award

I was informed July 16, 2009 by the following letter that I had been selected to receive the ACOG Distinguished Service Award to be presented May 19, 2010 at the annual clinical meeting in San Francisco:

Office of the Executive Vice President
Ralph W. Hale, MD, FACOG
Washington DC 20090-6920

Dear Dr. Sandmire:
I am pleased to tell you that the Executive Board of the American College of Obstetricians and Gynecologists has voted unanimously to present the ACOG Distinguished Service Award to you in recognition and appreciation of your outstanding contributions to the discipline of obstetrics and gynecology.

The College would like to have the privilege of presenting this award to you at its Presidential Inauguration and Convocation. This is to be held at 9:00 am on Wednesday, May 19, 2010, during the Annual Clinical Meeting of the College in San Francisco, CA. I do hope that it will be possible for you to attend. The dates of the meeting are May 15-19, 2010.

Sincerely, Ralph W. Hale, MD FACOG, Executive Vice President

Joining Sweetie and me to attend the Award Ceremony were son Kevin, daughter-in-law Karen, grandsons Kyle and Kurt, daughters Yvonne and Cheryl, daughter-in-law Beth and grandson Alec. The stay in San Francisco accompanied by family members was pleasant, the weather was perfect, and I felt humbled and honored to receive the national award.

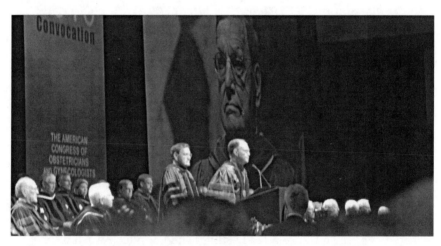

Receiving the American Congress of Obstetricians and Gynecologists Distinguished Service Award in San Francisco (May 19, 2010)

How do medical organizations choose the awardees from their up to 50,000 members? The answer is, it all begins at the local level with individuals recognizing the contributions of one of its members, documenting them and sending the nomination to, in my case, to the national ACOG executive board.

The two Wisconsin ACOG members responsible for my selection as the national ACOG Distinguished Service Award recipient were Drs. Donald Weber from EauClaire, Wisconsin and Dr. Robert Jaeger of Stevens Point, Wisconsin.

I was and still am humbled by being selected from a membership of 50,000 for this award. For that I owe a deep debt of gratitude to Don and Bob.

Wisconsin Association of Perinatal Care (WAPC)

In 1968, a group of obstetricians, including me, met with some leading Wisconsin pediatricians to plan for a new organization, the WAPC. The idea was to have an organization whose members were from different disciplines such as nurses, social workers and pharmacists as well as pediatricians and obstetricians. We had a few "hot tub" planning sessions at the Pioneer Inn in Oshkosh during 1968 and 1969. The organization became a reality early in the year 1970. I became a founding member and attended every meeting except for 2009. During my 41 years as a member I presented eight papers at the WAPC annual meetings.

Conway Periscope Interview (1999)

The Periscope is the quarterly news letter published by WAPC. The Winter 1999 issue contained the contents of an interview of me by Ann Conway in the Member Spotlight section. It represented my beliefs and thoughts at that time and is reproduced here in its entirety.

Herb Sandmire and his wife Crystal have attended every Annual Meeting since the inception of WAPC in 1970. Even before then, Herb was one of the core groups of leaders who met periodically at the Pioneer Inn in Oshkosh to plan the goals and purposes of WAPC. Herb currently has a practice limited to gynecologic care, though he practiced OB-GYN care in Green Bay since 1959.

Q. How did you come to choose a career in Medicine?
A. Becoming a doctor was an accident. I had an average scholastic high school record. My mother, who was a school teacher, encouraged me to go to UW-Platteville to major in agriculture education. I convinced her to let me try the UW-Madison. I entered the College of Agriculture and got interested in chemistry. When I changed my major to chemistry my classmates were all in pre-med, so I again changed my major to pre-med. I did not tell my parents that I had changed my major until I was accepted into Medical School in my junior year at the University.

Q. How did you choose OB-GYN as a specialty?

A. That was another accident. In 1954, when I was a Captain in the Air Force, I was stationed in Fairbanks, Alaska. Within one year after I completed my internship, at the age of 25, I was Chairman of the Department of OB-GYN at the base hospital. When I finished my military experience I realized that what I knew best was OB-GYN, so I went into a residency at the University of Iowa in Iowa City. In 1959 I entered into a partnership with a man who had been in solo practice in Green Bay, Dr. Stephen Austin.

Q. Describe your philosophy of medicine

A. A good doctor has three characteristics – good patient care, an interest in research and an interest in teaching. During my career I have been committed to all three. Good patient care is based on evidence-based medicine. We can provide better OB care by giving up some of the technology and interventions that do not benefit the patients. Since the 70s the public has been led to believe that more technology such as continuous fetal monitoring and ultrasound was better care. Through constant questioning and investigations I work to limit testing and interventions for patients to those that have proven benefits.

People who are in community hospitals have opportunities to do quality research, though it may have to be self-funded. My partner, Dr. DeMott, and I funded the statistical analysis of the four-part Green Bay Cesarean Section Study. This was an important effort to help answer the question of what is the right rate of Cesarean section.

I have been involved in educating medical students since the mid1960s and residents since 1980. I have a joint appointment with the University of Wisconsin Department of OB-GYN and the Department of Family Medicine and Practice. I had 20 years experience being a preceptor to senior medical students. I work with family practice residents and physicians in practice from all over the country who come to our visiting fellowship program for 2-4 weeks.

Q. What are the major issues to which you are paying attention?

A. An issue related to evidence-based practice, that I have a strong interest in, is reducing legal pressures that influence patient management. Ordering a lot of unnecessary tests that result in false positive results which then lead to more interventions, each with its own complications. Medical decisions should be based on the patient's best interest.

I work to minimize decision-making based on defensive medicine by being an "expert witness" for providers. In 1981, I was called as an expert witness in the case of an obstetrician practicing in Green Bay. From that point on I was asked to review 10-12 claims a year. Through published articles I gained national attention and now I am involved in claims around the country. In February, I will be involved in three cases – two local cases and one in Florida.

Q. What has changed your practice over the past years?

A. Antibiotics revolutionized all of medical practice, including OB-GYN practice. The unraveling of the Rh problem is a wonderful story. First we discovered the cause, then we learned to treat with exchange transfusions, and now we can prevent the condition with medication. The discovery of DNA led to the use of amniocentesis for genetic reasons. The development of ultrasound for the diagnosis of placenta previa and multiple gestations was significant as was the ability to prevent the rubella syndrome with a vaccine.

I have a list of "advances" that weren't: In other words, they were shams. That list includes electronic fetal monitoring, ultrasound for most of the excuses for which it is done, a section rate of more than 20%, and subjecting all breech presentations to cesarean section.

Q. Is there truth to the rumor that you are retiring?

A. In 1996 I stopped seeing obstetrical patients. Now I see women for gynecologic care about 25 hours per week, do legal work about 10 hours a week and teach about 5 hours a week. I'll think about retiring when I'm older. I'll be 70 in April.

Q. How would you describe the benefits of membership in WAPC?

A. It is nice to work with professionals who have a broad view of perinatal care. WAPC is multidisciplinary. I get to talk to people who all make valuable, yet different contributions and all have a common objective – to be the best that we can be in taking care of women and newborns.

During the 2005 annual meeting, I received the Callon/Leonard Award, the plaque's inscription reading, "The award is the highest honor the Association bestows for outstanding efforts and contributions to your community, to your profession and to a broad segment of society."

Dr. Dennis T. Costakos gave his Callon-Leonard Award nomination speech during the annual banquet in 2005. The amazing thing about Dr. Costakos's words was his comprehensive knowledge and understanding of obstetrics while working in another specialty as a neonatologist and, indeed, his familiarity with our obstetric literature.

Callon-Leonard Nomination of Dr. Herb Sandmire
By Dennis T. Costakos, MD, FAAP,WAPC President 2000

It is a great honor to nominate Dr. Herb Sandmire, fellow WAPC member, for the 2005 Callon-Leonard award. Dr. Sandmire is an Obstetrician-Gynecologist who took care of his patients and their families. He also made it a priority to share many of the lessons he discovered in his many decades of medical practice in Wisconsin. In the circles I travel, Green Bay does not just mean learning about the accomplishments and love of the Green Bay Packers, but of Dr. Herb Sandmire: physician, teacher, husband and father.

Dr. Sandmire was a beacon of light in terms of asking how do we achieve good outcomes in a cost effective manner. Dr. Sandmire has studied practice variations and has been looking at obstetrical outcomes long before this was in vogue to do. His practice in Green Bay has been a leader in taking a fresh look at auscultation versus electronic fetal monitoring, operative delivery versus vaginal delivery variations and outcomes.

His published observations in his Green Bay study III, Falling cesarean birth rates without a formal curtailment program AJOG (1994);179:790-802, again found that higher cesarean rates did not result in better perinatal outcome, thus confirming the results of his 1990 and 1992 studies. His work has improved perinatal outcomes in Wisconsin and not just Green Bay.

His work on intermittent auscultation is just as impressive in that it underscores the bedside medical management and cost effectiveness in the setting of improving outcomes. His work showed that intermittent auscultation is simple, provides objective information, and appeals to many well-informed patients. In addition, when the collection of information not relevant to management decisions is eliminated, intermittent auscultation nursing requirements are no greater than with electronic fetal monitoring. Laboring patients should receive information on both intermittent auscultation and electronic fetal monitoring to enable them to make an informed choice of method for their intrapartum fetal assessment.

Considering that many places in the United States see a dwindling supply of doctors and midwives willing to deliver babies because of possible litigation and high malpractice premiums, his work concerning the causation of Erb's palsy being the expulsive labor forces resulting in the stretching of the involved nerves over which the birth attendant has no control, is the type of published research results that improves perinatal care in Wisconsin.

Dr. Sandmire's work comes up at formal and informal gatherings, whether I'm talking with a fellow WAPC member (Dr. Russell Kirby, or a Stanford professor, Dr. Maurice Druzin, or at the European Perinatal Conference, Helsinki, Finland, when the Dublin, Ireland group lectured on the importance of the Green Bay experience to 2000 attendees, of which only 25 were American division or department Chairs in Neonatal-Perinatal Medicine, and the rest from 14 European countries).

In fact, I cannot remember a single annual meeting where I did not learn a major lesson from Dr. Sandmire. This could be in the setting of retrieving Dr. Nigel Paneth, in the rain, at the Madison airport, or at a breakfast session he would give at the annual meeting. Dr. Sandmire has treated many patients in Wisconsin and patients who voted he should get this award in that his practice thrived because the patients thrived. WAPC has a special member and friend who has attended and participated in our wonderful organization over several decades in his early days of practice and now. Dr. Sandmire has made many medical and scientific innovations for the practice of perinatal medicine in Wisconsin and the Globe. Please honor him with the Leonard-Callon Award for his life time of hard work, sacrifice, dedication, innovation and love of his Wisconsin patients and families.

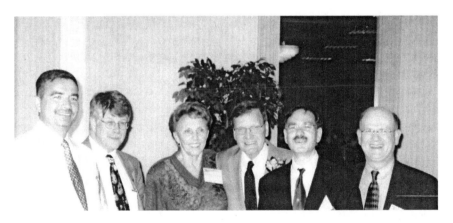

After receiving the WAPC 2005 Callon/Leonard Award. From left to right: Philip Nielsen, Russ Kirby, Sweetie,Me,Dennis Costakos and Don Weber

ACOG District VI

My partner, the late Dr. Austin, attended most of the national ACOG meetings, and I was an active participant in ACOG District VI meetings.

On a September day in 1958, I traveled from my residency duties at the University of Iowa to Des Moines, Iowa, the site of ACOG District VI annual meeting. My paper, entitled "Ectopic Pregnancy: A review of 182 cases," received the "First Place Residents' Papers Award."

The ACOG District VI meeting in November of 1960 was held in Chicago, Illinois, where I delivered a paper entitled "Prevention and treatment of postpartum hemorrhage." In November of 1963, I delivered a paper entitled "Office gynecological surgery" at the District VI meeting in Milwaukee.

In November 1970, at the ACOG District VI meeting in St. Paul, Minnesota, I delivered a paper that received worldwide attention entitled "Experience with 15,000 consecutive pap smears." (discussed elsewhere) The main conclusion of my study was that birth control pills did not increase the risk for cervical cancer, contrary to a report from a New York study.

The September 1985 meeting of District VI was held in Milwaukee, and my paper there was entitled "Fertility after IUD discontinuation."

In September of 1986, the District VI meeting was held in Winnipeg, Manitoba, Canada. "Shoulder dystocia: Its incidence and associated risk factors" was the title of my presentation. This represents my first research and paper regarding my more recent interest in shoulder dystocia and brachial plexus injury. Our first District VI meeting in Winnipeg was in 1962. The meetings in Winnipeg were close enough for us to drive, so we combined a little family time with the trip. Each time we took two of our children with us. I remember how very hospitable the Canadians were. One of the obstetricians even hired a baby sitter at his home for our children and his.

At the September 1989 St. Paul, Minnesota District VI meeting, I presented two papers, the first entitled "Exposing the causation of cerebral palsy myths," and the second called "Electronic fetal monitoring".

ACOG District VI meeting in London, September 12-21, 2003

The ACOG District VI met in London, England for their annual 2003 meeting. Since we had not travelled to London previously, we went early for sightseeing before the meeting began and stayed beyond for a few days.

Prior to the meeting we had a bus ride to Bath and stayed in the Bath Spa Hotel that Winston Churchill frequented during World War II. The hotel is situated on huge, landscaped grounds and is quite elegant. In fact, the government took it over during the war. England is very pretty, and we actually had great sunny, warm weather for September. After checking in, we walked around the very pretty little city. We saw the apartment where Jane Austen lived, and our guide gave us some interesting history of the place.

The next day we went to Stratford-upon-Avon and toured Shakespeare's birthplace and Anne Hathaway's cottage which really was a quite a large home for that time. The little villages we rode through were Stow-on-the-Wold, Moreton-in-Marsh and Chipping Camden, where we saw the attractive Cotswold homes. These little towns were very clean and attractive. The next day we saw more of the city Bath, touring the Roman Baths before heading back to London. Along the way, we stopped at Stonehenge.

Back in London, we walked around the city near our hotel and found a restaurant where we celebrated our fifty second wedding anniversary. My meeting started the next day, but the afternoons were always free for other activities. We saw "Mamma Mia!" at the Prince Edward Theatre and had a great Italian dinner near the theatre.

Sweetie attended a group breakfast at Harrods which was scheduled for our spouses. Inside the store, she saw the Memorial to the late British Princess Diana and her Egyptian lover, Dodi Fayed, whose father is the store's owner. At the end of breakfast, our spouses were given a shoppers' tour of the building. My wife enjoyed seeing members of her group buying overpriced stuff at Harrods.

The next day we had a tour of Windsor Castle, the official residence of Queen Elizabeth II, followed by dinner with our whole group at an English Pub called the Prospect of Whitby. This Pub is London's oldest (established in 1520), riverside pub near Greenwich.

We got to see the Tower of London, the famous London Eye, Westminster Abbey and Buckingham Palace when we toured more of London. As we walked through the streets, our guide pointed out the apartment building where William and Harry stayed when in the area. Of course, there was a guard posted at the entry.

The weather cooperated so we could do lots of walking. I remarked that they read and write English here but I do not understand the language they speak!! Our ten-day obligatory trip to England was indeed a very interesting time, and we were glad we went.

The Central Association Obstetricians Gynecologists (CAOG)

CAOG is a prestigious organization with membership limited to 500 invitees from 28 central states. I was sponsored by professors from Iowa and Wisconsin and became a member in 1972. The new members each year were required to present a paper at the following annual meeting. This requirement demonstrated the desire of the Association to emphasize the production of high-caliber research. Through an arrangement with the *American Journal of Obstetrics and Gynecology (AJOG)*, papers presented at the CAOG annual meeting were automatically submitted to *AJOG* with a high percentage being accepted for publication.

My participation in CAOG entailed serving on the Board of Trustees from 1983 to 1986 and serving on the nominating committee. During my membership in CAOG, I presented 13 papers at the annual meetings, all of which were subsequently published in the prestigious *AJOG*.

My first paper in 1973, at Scottsdale, Arizona, was required by my becoming a member the prior year, and the title was "Curettage as an office procedure." It was subsequently published in the May issue of *AJOG*.

Two years later, we journeyed to Colorado Springs to deliver a paper concerning our research entitled "Carcinoma of the cervix in oral contraceptive steroid and IUD users and non-users."

Traveling to Biloxi, Mississippi in 1977, I gave a paper on the recent research I had begun entitled "Minilaparotomy tubal sterilization." The focus of this research was to develop a procedure that could compete with the laparoscopic procedure but with markedly less risk of vascular or intestinal complications.

My next presentation, in 1981, was the result of my establishing the Green Bay Surgical Center in January of 1978. The meeting again took place in Scottsdale, and my presentation was "Discussion of a free-standing surgical unit: A success or failure?"

We traveled to Detroit for the 1984 annual meeting and renewed our acquaintance with Marty and Jean Daitch, our colleagues from our Air Force Alaska experience. Our paper (co-authored with my partner Dr. Bob Cavanaugh) was entitled "Long-term use of intrauterine devices in a private practice." We were humbled when this paper was selected for the "Community Hospital Award."

We drove down to Milwaukee for the 1986 meeting. Because of an epidemic of medical law suits, my paper on shoulder dystocia became a

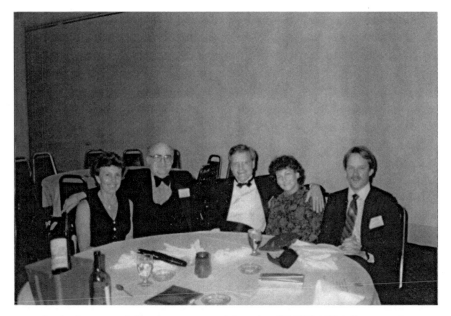

At the banquet following our receiving the CAOG 1984 Community Hospital Award in Detroit. Also present are co-author R. Cavanaugh and our friends from our 1954-56 Alaskan days, Dr. and Mrs. Marty Daitch

new interest of mine. The presentation was entitled "Discussion of shoulder dystocia: A fetal/physician risk."

In the mid-1980s, the nation's cesarean section birth rate escalated to 20 to 25 percent, up from five percent in 1970. Clearly, this increase could not be justified on the basis of anatomical or physiological changes in pregnant women. Women's pelvises did not shrink nor did babies' head sizes increase. This unbelievable increase could only be explained by physicians' change in practice style. Dr. DeMott and I planned a four-part research project in an attempt to discover the reasons for the cesarean birth increase and ways it could be reversed.

The first of three papers was presented at the CAOG annual meeting in 1989. Its title was "The Green Bay cesarean section study I: The Physician factor as a determinant of cesarean birth rates." Our conclusions were that higher cesarean rates did not result in better neonatal outcomes, that physician practice style was the only apparent determinant of the increased rates for the eleven obstetricians studied, and that current cesarean rates could be substantially reduced without sacrificing newborn safety.

Our second paper, entitled "The Green Bay cesarean section study II: The physician factor as a determinant of cesarean birth rates for failed labor," concluded that a cesarean rate reduction program for patients for non-progressive labor would be successful if it included more oxytocin for more patients for longer periods of time and if physicians waited until more advanced cervical dilatation is achieved before the administration of oxytocin.

At the 1992 CAOG annual meeting I presented "A discussion of reducing cesarean births at a primarily private university hospital." Our third cesarean paper, entitled "The Green Bay cesarean section study III: Falling cesarean birth rates without a formal curtailment program" argued that relatively low cesarean rates could be reduced further without sacrificing newborn safety, that cesarean rates could be further reduced without a formal curtailment program, and that optimal and achievable cesarean rates in the Green Bay community appeared to be in the seven to eight percent range. Our fourth research study was not presented at the CAOG, but published in the *AJOG* in 1996. Its title was "The Green Bay cesarean section study IV: The physician factor as a determinant of cesarean birth rates for the large fetus." In it we concluded that patients with a suspected macrosomic (large) fetus should be given the same opportunity to achieve a normal delivery as patients with smaller fetuses.

In 1998, at the meeting in Kansas City, I provided a "Discussion of obstetrician characteristics on cesarean delivery rates: A community hospital experience."

In Washington, D.C. in 2004, I provided a "Discussion of the accuracy of estimated fetal weight in shoulder dystocia and traumatic birth injury." Finally, in 2008, I made my last presentation at the CAOG meeting in New Orleans. Its title was "Brachial plexus injury causation: What are the controversies?"

Society for the advancement of contraception (SAC)

My membership in this organization began at its meeting in Chicago in 1986, where I presented a paper entitled "Fertility after intrauterine device (IUD) discontinuation" – later published in *Advances in Contraception*. In October of the following year, Crystal and I attended the meeting in Caracas, Venezuela. At the conclusion of that meeting, we took a little side trip to Margarita Island, a short flight off the coast of Venezuela. The advantage of our membership in SAC was that it took us around the world to places we would not have otherwise visited.

In November of 1990, we attended the SAC meeting in Singapore, a beautiful Asian city-state with strict rules regarding personal conduct – a $500 fine for littering, for example. This was not a problem for us, since we had no intention of littering in this beautiful city or anywhere else.

We visited the museum that depicted the historic signing of the defeat of the British by the Japanese Empire early in World War II. At the Singapore meeting, we met and exchanged ideas with a few Scandinavian gynecologists and thereafter corresponded with one of them. In addition, we became acquainted with Dr. Jennifer Wilson from New Zealand, who shared a common interest with me and presented a paper, as I had previously, entitled "A New Zealand study of fertility after IUD use." Two years later, while we were traveling to Melbourne, Australia for my expert witness testimony, Jennifer arranged a reception for us with her and her New Zealand colleagues during our stop-over in their country (small world).

While in Singapore, we took the elevator to the deck on the 71st floor of the Westin Stamford (the world's highest hotel) and had a Singapore sling, to overcome our fear of heights, followed by dinner at the Compass Rose restaurant, also on the 71st floor. Sweetie, not being accustomed to alcoholic beverages and the altitude, became a little goofy, or perhaps *goofier*, that night. Another highlight was having dinner in the restaurant in the world famous Raffles Hotel.

A side boat trip to Indonesia provided interesting sight-seeing for these two American tourists. Another boat trip to Sanatosa Island with return by cable car provided fantastic views from a high altitude.

Our next attended SAC meeting was late in October of 1992 in Barcelona, Spain. We combined a self-planned vacation tour of Spain before the meeting without any prior reservations – stopping along the way when we felt like it. Now, 18 years later, it is hard to believe how fearless we were. Actually, we only had to worry about finding a hotel one afternoon with a rental car on the way back to the airport in Madrid after the meeting was over. We ultimately found a small hotel just before darkness set in.

Our 16-day trip entailed multiple methods of travel. We landed in Madrid, went by bus to Segovia, by fast train to Seville, stopping in Cordoba along the way, by bus to Algeciras on Costa Del Sol, saw the Rock of Gibraltar, and went along the coast by bus to Malaga where we got a train up the East coast to Barcelona. We covered a lot of miles and many stops, including the sites of Expo 92 in Seville and the Olympics in Barcelona (both of which had just finished). I think all of

Spain was cleaned and polished for those events, and we reaped the benefits. It was also the 500th anniversary of Christopher Columbus coming to America.

While in Barcelona we saw the God of Fertility statue, the Picasso museum, the Bull Ring, and the yet unfinished Gaudi structure.

The last SAC meeting we attended was in Guatemala City, Guatemala, Central America from March 7th to the 10th, 1995. The highlight of our days in Guatemala was the Antigua tour where we saw ruins from the earthquake of 1774, a large Jade factory, and the famously described "scenery where time seems to have stood still in the colonial era." "Cobblestone streets, whitewashed walls, flowers in constant bloom, and centuries-old arcades [gave us] something to remember forever."

We did have one scare when our credit card was missing following lunch at the Camino Real Hotel. We became aware that it was missing and promptly alerted Visa to cancel the card. Apparently, we had left the restaurant before the waitress returned our card. Anyway, all is well that ends well.

During the latter part of the 1990s, the high U.S. cesarean rate was receiving increasing attention in academic centers. I was asked to provide a report of the Green Bay cesarean study (four separate published papers) at two separate national programs, both entitled *Safely Reducing Cesarean Rates*. The first, sponsored by Cambridge Health Resources, took place at the Fairmont Copley Plaza in Boston on June eighth and ninth, 1998. The second national meeting, sponsored by AIC World-wide, was held at the Caribe Royal in Orlando, Florida, May third and fourth, 1999.

The focus of my presentations was to describe techniques used in Green Bay, Wisconsin to reduce cesarean rates without sacrificing new-born or maternal outcomes.

Red Cross Board of Directors, Lakeland Chapter 1975 to 1981

I enjoyed the six years I served on the Red Cross board. I found other board members, the Red Cross staff, and the director to be caring, productive, competent individuals dedicated to their work. There was one exception, an individual who presumed it was his responsibility to adjust the "bra" of a female co-worker. He was summarily given the pink slip by the director on the basis that he was creating a hostile work environment.

A short time later, a sheriff appeared at my office to deliver a summons based on the "bra-adjuster's" lawsuit against the Red Cross and its directors for firing him with insufficient cause. Unbelievably, a few of my co-board members thought we should offer him a small sum to be free of the lawsuit. **I SAID "HELL NO" TO THAT IDEA.** The suit was ultimately dropped, but "the bra adjuster" continued his harassment of the director by bumping into the back of his car as he was going home from work. His true character came out a year or two later when he was caught stealing sausages from a grocery store.

CHAPTER 28

The Hawaiian connection

IN THE FALL of 1984, Sweetie and I travelled to Maui to attend the annual meeting of District VI American College of Obstetricians and Gynecologists (ACOG). While at the banquet, a beautiful Hawaiian girl went through the crowd looking for novice hula dancers to train on the spot. As she made her way toward our table, our friends motioned to her to select me to join her on stage. My brief moment in the limelight included some rudimentary talent, by my own assessment at least. This early performance would foreshadow another glorious display of choreography 20 years later when, on vacation in Punta Cana, Dominican Republic, I won the "Sexiest Man" contest – recorded in the annals of history by a certificate I received from the Master of Ceremonies. I had tied with my grandson Kyle in the pre-liminary scoring, forcing a final dance - off to determine the winner.

At the conclusion of our meeting on Maui, we travelled to Kauai and then on to Honolulu, where we visited the Pearl Harbor Museum.

In January of 1986, Sweetie, sons Mike and Dave, and I returned to Maui to attend the third annual meeting of the Society of Law and Medicine. Over the ensuing years I have attended all of their annual meetings except for 2010 and will be going again in January of 2011. It is an excellent meeting to advance my knowledge and skills in the med-ical legal aspects of obstetrics. In addition, it provides an opportunity to meet obstetricians and lawyers who have similar interests. Aubrey Milunsky runs the whole program and always selects reliable speakers.

On that January 1986 afternoon, the day before we were to leave for home, we drove up the beautiful Kanapali coast, took some pictures on a bluff, and while focusing the camera, I said to Sweetie, Dave and Mike that we should build a condo for Sweetie on that very spot.

Although said in jest, we all agreed the idea had a nice ring to it.

Later that evening, while shopping for Hawaiian shirts, we learned of real estate agent Gloria Rose, who showed us some condos in South Maui before our return home the next afternoon.

Karen, Kevin, Sweetie and I returned in March 1986 and bought condominium 507 at the beautiful Polo Beach Club. In December of that year, our whole family spent our first Christmas season together on Maui. That same tradition continued on a regular basis for the next fourteen years and on an irregular basis thereafter.

In 1990 we bought condo 505 at the Polo Beach Club as well as the recently finished A 108, G 202, G 111 and I 117 at the Maui Kamaole condo complex. Two years later, we bought G 102 at Maui Kamaole on a resale basis.

We enjoyed staying at one of our condos and also at times sharing them with many guests. In March of 1992 there were 23 of us from Green Bay vacationing in our condos. This included members of three United Methodist bridge clubs. There were other times when we entertained fewer than 23, but still a substantial number of our friends. We have many fond memories of vacationing in Maui with these friends.

Sweetie assumed the role of CEO for "Crystal Condo Properties," a partnership with our five children formed in 1990. She had interesting exchanges from rental clients from all over the world, especially from Japan, the Scandinavian countries, Australia and Canada.

During the 1990s and early 2000s, we donated time in one of our condos to fund-raising auctions of charitable organizations and churches seven or eight times a year.

Finally, with the desire of CEO Sweetie to take "early" retirement at age 71, in 2002, we sold six of our seven condos. The remaining one (I 117 at Maui Kamaole) now belongs to our five children. They take care of all matters concerning the maintenance and renting of that condo. Sweetie and I are no longer partners in Crystal Condo Properties.

CHAPTER 29

Mid-life crisis???

IN 1986, STATE Senator Donald Hanaway became the Attorney General of Wisconsin, vacating his state senate seat. I decided that if I got a sufficient number of votes from health care personnel, I might have a chance of being elected. I formed a campaign committee of Green Bay leaders that included Bart and Cherry Starr. We developed a nice brochure and mailed out 5000 of them, but I did not ring doorbells. My personal campaigning involved participating in debates with three other candidates.

On Election Day, Crystal and I were the first two voters at our polling place, and on leaving I said to her, "At least I have two votes," to which she retorted, "Don't be too sure." As I reflect back on it 24 years later, I am glad that I did not win. Since losing in the senate race, I probably have accomplished more by continuing my obstetric career than I could have accomplished as a state senator. As usual, and looking back to that time period, Crystal was once again right about what was best for us.

The foes of women's rights increased their picketing from the usual six or so to fifty on February 11, 1987, hoping to discourage voters from supporting me. In response to the protestors, Kathleen McGillis, editor of the *Green Bay News Chronicle*, wrote the following editorial:

> *Green Bay News Chronicle*
> *Friday, February 15, 1987*
> **Clean teeth, dirty politics**
> *At long last, I got my teeth cleaned Thursday.*
> *Frantically brushing my teeth before the appointment I caught*
> *the noon news on the radio.*

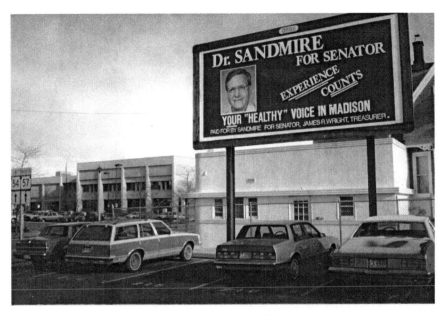

"Mid-life crisis." Sandmire for Senator (1987)

In making the date to visit my dentist in the Medical Arts Building about a month ago, I thought about the convenience of the office location – just a few blocks from where I live.

The news reminded me of the reasons many of the people in town know where the Medical Arts Building is – Herb Sandmire also has an office there.

If you haven't heard of Dr. Sandmire, you've been breezing past The News-Chronicle editorial, and local news pages.

A bevy of letters have appeared in protest of Sandmire's candidacy for the Republican nomination to the 2nd district race.

Sandmire is said to perform abortions. And Thursday, my dental appointment day of all days, about 50 people showed up to protest outside the Bellin Building.

A variety of scenarios reeled through my head before I left the house: an angry mob, harassing anyone going into the building. "Baby killer," they would shout at me, a young woman with dirty teeth.

As it turned out, the most troubling image by the building was parked kitty-corner from the building when I walked up – a Green Bay police car.

The car and the four remaining marchers there when I entered the building were still there when I exited 90 minutes later.

Cavityless! But the whole thing made me mad. I don't know Dr. Sandmire, and I'll probably vote Democrat. But it digs at me that he should be somewhat terrorized – not to mention everyone else in the building – for allegedly performing abortions.

Perhaps it's just a matter of how each of us defines campaign issues and who is eligible for questioning on which issue.

Has anyone asked the other candidates if they, their wife or lover has ever had an abortion?

Or if they regularly lie, steal, cheat, are unfaithful or covet their neighbor's VCR?

Or if they believe in God or are gay?

Or aren't those campaign issues either?

This editorial prompted several letters to the editor attacking Ms. McGillis. A typical example:

Readers comment
February 21, 1987
Green Bay News Chronicle
McGillis and her ilk

In response to Ms. McGillis's column of February 13. I would like to ask Ms. McGillis this question. Have you ever given any thought to the fact that perhaps the police were across from the Medical Arts Building to insure the safety of the marchers from paranoid people like yourself.

Through the years pro-lifers have endured much bigotry, hatred, ridicule, and paranoia exhibited toward us. We have also encountered and endured verbal as well as physical abuse. Does Ms. McGillis really believe that what a reporter from a small newspaper has to say will discourage us from continuing our fight for the rights of the helpless? You see, Ms. McGillis, we are always prepared for the onslaught of intolerance by people like yourself. How can we get it through to you and others that we have every right to express our views as do the "Freezenicks," "Greenpeace," "unions". And even journalists, etc.

You and your ilk spout the same pattern of rhetoric, which leads me to believe you are paranoid.

You and your ilk's relentless attacks on pro-lifers' free expression speech rights pose a very real terrorist threat to our society and has chilling ramifications. There is such ugliness in bigotry.

May I give you a little lesson in geography, Ms. McGillis? The terrorism takes place inside the Medical Arts Building, not outside.

How can you state that an abortionist is being terrorized by being publically picketed because of his barbaric actions, and not see that he terrorizes a child every time he stills the heartbeat of that child?

Stick to the issue, Ms. McGillis. And killing of helpless unborn children is the issue.

Where is your intelligence, for heaven's sake? If a doctor was raping women in the Medical Arts Building, would you put him in the same category as with someone who is stealing, lying, cheating, or covets his neighbor's VCR? I repeat, stick the issue, it makes for better journalism. – Mrs. M. F. Williquette, 1512 St. George St., Green Bay, WI 54302.

Francis Kamenick, the only individual who repeatedly picketed at our home, wrote this heartfelt letter to me:

October 8, 1989, Sunday afternoon
Francis Kamenick
1317 South Oneida
Green Bay, Wisconsin 54304
Dear Doctor Sandmire,
I thought you deserved an explanation of who I am, (You were nice enough to identify yourself in a civil manner).
I am Francis Kamenick, the Man who picketed in front of your house this afternoon, with the red flag.
I come in peace. I mean no harm to you or your family. Peace be to you.
My fervent hope is that my peaceful picketing in front of your home may help you realize what you are doing to your, as well as mine, brothers and sisters, who are not born yet. For surely these innocents are your brothers and sisters, as well as mine. I hope you will come to see this, as Doctor Nathanson did. (A former abortionist who reportedly operated the largest abortion clinic on the East coast.)
These are your own brothers and sisters you are killing, Dr. Sandmire.
All Doctors know <u>all</u> life begins at Conception, and that includes Human Life. The genetic union between two human beings can only result in Human Life. Surely all doctors know this.
I come to you, not to judge you, (That is up to God.) but to appeal to you, as your <u>brother</u>, to stop the killing of my unborn brothers and sisters.
My own mother told me you were always known as a fine baby doctor, and that you could get women pregnant where other doctors had failed. My mother graduated from St. Mary's school of nursing

in 1936, I was born 1938. My mother claimed you would often ask her to "Special" a baby case for you, (she always loved babys.) just as you were known as the "baby" doctor. She said she could never understand why you turned to abortion. Doctor Kelley of old St. Mary's hospital delivered me.

My mother told me how you had a "special" way with children that no other doctor had.

My mother always had a special regard for you, and the cases she "specialed" for you. Her name was "Naomi" Kamenick, she was a short chunky nurse who often worked for Dr. Kelley in old St. Mary's hospital, and later: she was a supervisor at the new St Vincent hospital. She always had a kindly smile on her face, Hi. She always loved babys [sic] and life.

I applaud your kind attitude toward us picketers when we picketed the Medical Arts building 3 years ago 300 strong. You strongly defended our right to picket, saying we were only exercising our "American Right" as Americans. I deeply appreciate this.

Later, that night, at your reception at the Riverside ballroom, you came out to meet us (5 picketers.) You kindly introduced yourself and your wife and shook hands with each and everyone of us, and invited us in to your reception. We of course refused, if for no other reason we thought it would look like surrender, if we laid our picket signs down, and walked into the hall. (I had the red flag.) I was surprised you would shake hands with us, and invite us in to your own reception.

I am impressed with your warm and outgoing personality; you seem to be a man who is willing to look at both sides of an issue. God Love you.

Sincerely yours,
Francis Kamenick

CHAPTER 30

$\mathcal{JUD}$ Research

AS A CONTINUATION of my research on the use of the intrauterine contraceptive device (IUD), as previously stated, I presented a paper entitled "Long-term use of the intrauterine contraceptive device in private practice" at the 52nd annual meeting of CAOG in Detroit, Michigan on October 12, 1984. Co-author Cavanaugh and I were presented with the CAOG Community Hospital Paper Award at the meeting. The paper was subsequently published in the May 15, 1985 issue of *The American Journal of Obstetrics and Gynecology*.

The objectives of this research were to compare the Lippes Loop, Dalkon Shield and CU-7 IUDs for pregnancy rates and the frequency of pelvic inflammatory disease (PID). Our findings revealed no differences in the pregnancy rates for the three types of IUDs and no differences in PID frequency between the Dalkon shield and the CU-7 device.

Professor R. David Miller, University of California Irvine, in an unsolicited letter, praised our research findings as indicated in his following letter:

> *University of California, Irvine*
> *Department of Obstetrics and Gynecology*
> *January 30, 1985*
> *Herbert F. Sandmire, M. D. FACOG*
> *201 St. Mary's Blvd*
> *Green Bay, Wisconsin 54301*
> *Dear Dr. Sandmire:*
> *I would like to congratulate you on your presentation on the comparison of long-term IUD use in a private practice population. This*

study, in my opinion is a singular landmark study as it is the first, to the best of my knowledge dealing with a "real world population" as opposed to a high-risk hospital based population.

In the event that you are able, I would be delighted to invite you to speak at UCI on your findings. We obviously would cover your cost of getting here as well as providing an honorarium.

In the interim, I would appreciate a copy of the abstract and any additional data which you would be willing to share at this time. I feel the aspects of your study have a very important bearing on how we approach the problem of IUD's with medical students. I am sure you are aware of the fact that at this time we rely almost solely on hospital data which, to say the least, is a highly selected population.

I look forward to hearing from you in the near future.

Sincerely,

R. David Miller, M.D.

Associate Professor and Director

Div of Ob/Gyn Infectious Disease

Coordinator of Grand Rounds

Meanwhile, the Dalkon Shield had been pulled off the market by the Robins Company in the mid-1970s following many patient lawsuits alleging that it caused PID. The suits were combined into a single class action suit. Prior to the beginning of the single class action activity, the Robins Company had settled about 60 individual lawsuits. The Robins Company, when faced with an overwhelming number of suits, declared bankruptcy, and the Federal Bankruptcy Court was to establish "fair" compensation for each of the persons filing a complaint.

I was chosen by the Robins Company to be their consultant and chief expert witness, presumably because of our published, award-winning paper. I worked with the late Carol Hewitt from Portland, Oregon, lead counsel for the company (this association ultimately led to our son Michael joining Ms. Hewitt's law firm). This involved trips to Portland, Los Angeles, Richmond, Virginia and Chicago to prepare the best position possible for the company. We developed a seven-class hierarchy of injuries according to the requirements dictated by the bankruptcy judge and based on the company's prior settlements. In addition, the company was not allowed to use any scientific advances developed since the time of the company's settlements several years earlier. This was severely detrimental to the company, preventing it from requiring claimants to submit to the recently developed chlamydia test. Chlamydia is a common sexually transmitted disease and the number one cause of tubal infertility. So much for the goal of our civil justice system that supposedly is to "search for the truth." The plaintiff's committee was seeking seven billion in payments, while the company and its stockholders were holding out for under two billion.

My six-hour deposition was taken by Attorney Wendell B. Alcorn, Jr., of Cadwalader, Wickersham and Taft law firm in New York, at the Hyatt Regency O'Hare in Chicago, on October 28, 1987. On November 6, 1987, I testified for five hours in Federal Court in Richmond, Virginia, on behalf of the Robins Company. Crystal and I were treated like the Queen and King of England in Richmond, put up in a fancy hotel in a suite with four rooms and three bathrooms, each with its own phone. Crystal got into a little trouble at the hearing by sitting in the seat apparently reserved for the Robins Company's in-house counsel.

A little humor came out during my testimony when Attorney Alcorn, the prominent New York law firm partner, after giving me a long hypothetical scenario and asking for my agreement (which I couldn't give), repeated the same over again and asked for my agreement (which I didn't give him), and then asked, "Where did I go wrong?" I answered, "I DON'T KNOW." My answer resulted in an immediate murmur from the more than 400 lawyers present in the courtroom that was loud enough to awaken the judge who asked the bailiff, "What did he say?" The bailiff responded, "HE SAID I DON'T KNOW." *(The little known obstetrician from small town Green Bay left the interrogating lawyer danglingly "wrong" before a courtroom packed with lawyers)*.

Portions of my testimony were reported in the *Richmond Times-Dispatch*, the *Richmond News Leader*, the *New York Times*, and the *Washington Post*. Excerpts from the *New York Times* and *Washington Post* include the following:

New York Times, Saturday, November 7, 1987:

Testimony on Robins Continues; session set for weekend

Today's testimony came after attorneys for Robins and the claimants met Thursday night at the insistence of Judge Merhige but once again failed to bridge their differences. It is generally assumed among lawyers who have packed the court room here that Judge Merhige wants to see a larger fund than the company has proposed.

Dr. Herbert F. Sandmire, a Green Bay, Wisconsin obstetrician and gynecologist called by Robins as an expert witness, argued that a venereal disease that was not identified when the Dalkon shield was introduced in 1971 was responsible for many of the infertility problems blamed on IUDs.

Dr. Sandmire said that when studies separated out monogamous women, who were less likely to catch sexually transmitted diseases, from those with multiple partners, IUD users showed no greater infertility than the general population.

Dr. Sandmire also disagreed with studies that suggest an increased level of ectopic pregnancies could be blamed on Dalkon shield use.

Washington Post, Sunday, November 8, 1987:

Experts at Hearing Dispute IUD Safety

On Friday, Dr. Herbert F. Sandmire, a medical witness for Robins, cited a new report by Lee in which he said, Lee had refined the study data to isolate IUD users in stable, monogamous unions. She found "little appreciable risk" of PID in those women compared to women using no contraception, Sandmire said.

Today, Kessel echoed Sandmire's testimony.

Kessel said he was "impressed by the reevaluation" Lee had made and gave the shield along with other IUDs a ringing endorsement for safety.

Judge Robert Merhige, Jr., issued his ruling on December 13, 1987 requiring the Robins Company to set up a trust fund of $2.4 billion dollars to compensate for past and future injuries. Interestingly, a certain number of "injured" persons declined to accept the trust's offer and reentered the civil justice system. This was a bad decision on their part because they no longer had the previously described restrictions that applied to the Robins Company by Judge Merhige Jr., and the company's lawyers were able to require chlamydia testing, all of which were positive for the eight cases for which I was an expert witness. Naturally, we received a defense verdict in all of those cases, and the claimants received nothing.

This whole Dalkon Shield saga was farcical in its masquerading as a legitimate "seeking of the truth" while at the same time Judge Merhige Jr. was erecting barriers to the discovery of the truth.

My testimony for the Robins Company was strengthened by some of my own research. I presented a paper entitled "Fertility after IUD discontinuation" at the annual meeting of ACOG District VI on September 27, 1985 in Milwaukee and at the annual meeting of the Society for the Advancement of Contraception (SAC) in Chicago on September 26, 1986. It was published in *Advances in Contraception* on November 6, 1986. A further presentation with the same title occurred on June 3, 1988 at the Debrecen Medical College in Debrecen, Hungary and on June 10, 1988 at the Warsaw Medical College in Warsaw, Poland.

CHAPTER 31

Adolescent Pregnancy Prevention Services Board

IN THE SPRING of 1987, I was appointed by newly elected Wisconsin Governor Tommy Thompson to the Adolescent Pregnancy Prevention Services Board. Regarding a woman's legal right to have an abortion, the board consisted of three pro-choice and three anti-choice members. Our main responsibility was to award grants from state funds to various programs designed to reduce or prevent adolescent pregnancies. During my three-year appointment, I attended five to six meetings a year at the State Capitol building. At our November 3, 1987 meeting, we approved a grant for Rosalie Manor of $41,925. The *Milwaukee Journal* described our meeting follows:

> **State grant OK'd for Rosalie Manor, by Charles E. Friederich**
>
> *Madison, Wis. – A sharply divided state board approved a grant of $41,925 to Rosalie Manor, a Catholic-operated teen pregnancy program in Milwaukee, on Tuesday.*
>
> *The long-delayed grant was approved on a 4-2 vote of the State Adolescent Pregnancy Prevention Services Board. The board majority decided that, although Rosalie Manor was sponsored by a Catholic order, its teen pregnancy program was non-sectarian and thus could qualify for state funds.*
>
> *The board, which allocates state pregnancy funds, is made up of three opponents of abortion and three pro-choice members. All three anti-abortion members voted for the grant to Rosalie: two of the three pro-choice members voted against it. The swing vote was that of Her-*

bert F. Sandmire, a Green Bay obstetrician and gynecologist and pro-choice member of the board. He voted for the grant saying he was convinced that Rosalie Manor's services "would not be religiously influenced."

Sister Rosemarie Fischer, the agency's director, told board members before Tuesday's vote that Rosalie Manor was governed by a non-sectarian board.

"I could not tell you what the religious affiliation of our board members and members of our staff is," she said.

Charles Phillips, a board member and executive director of the Wisconsin Catholic Conference, slammed his fist on the table at one point and accused the board's pro-choice members of trying to block a grant that, he said, met the board's own standards.

On the 9 th and 10th of May 1988, our board sponsored a two-day meeting at the Madison Sheraton Hotel entitled "Preventing teen pregnancy: Problems and Solutions." I delivered a lecture entitled "Health services for teens."

CHAPTER 32

Cerebral Palsy

IN THE MIDDLE of the 1970s, physicians in general and obstetricians specifically were facing a litigation epidemic. The cost of liability insurance increased from $10,000 to $30,000/year over a three to four year time period and peaked at $60,000/year in the 1990s.

The main allegation involved in lawsuits against obstetricians was that labor was mismanaged, the fetus was receiving insufficient oxygen and earlier delivery would have prevented the resultant cerebral palsy (CP). As I stated earlier, my first experience as an expert witness was helping defend Green Bay obstetrician Dr. Utrie in the Tisch case filed in 1980, with a defense verdict in 1983. Plaintiff's attorney James Murphy asked the appeals court to reverse the circuit court defense verdict, but was unsuccessful in that effort in 1985. From the 1980s to the mid-1990s, I helped defend obstetricians in more than 150 cases, most of which involved allegations that the physician failed to prevent CP.

The experience I had as an expert witness helping obstetricians who were sued and my resultant literature review on CP led to my first presentation on this topic at the July 1986 annual meeting of the Wisconsin Society of Obstetrics and Gynecology, entitled "Cerebral palsy: What are the causes?"

Recognizing the need to educate physicians, nurses and attorneys, I was the organizer and program director of a multidisciplinary symposium entitled "Cerebral Palsy: Is it preventable?" held at the Holiday Inn in Oshkosh, Wisconsin on July 16, 1987. Amazingly, we received support from several sponsors, including the Wisconsin Society of Obstetrics and Gynecology, Wisconsin Association of Perinatal Care, United Cerebral Palsy of Wisconsin, Inc., Wisconsin Division of Health: Family and Community Health Services, Maternal and Child's

Health, and the Wisconsin Department of Public Instruction's Bureau of Children with Physical Needs. Symposium Funding Support came from the Wisconsin Division of Health, Physicians Insurance Company of Wisconsin, and the Wisconsin Society of Obstetrics and Gynecology.

The next challenge was to obtain outstanding speakers, all of whom were experts in their respective disciplines. Here again, the response was terrific, with not a single refusal from any of the six I had chosen. The outstanding speakers, each with a national reputation, included the late Paul Grimstad, attorney from Manitowoc, Wisconsin and one of the best defense attorneys in our state; Maureen Hack, M.B., Ch.B., Director of the High Risk Follow-up program at Case Western Reserve University's Rainbow Babies and Children's Hospital in Cleveland, Ohio; Sandra Kramer, J.D., attorney with the law firm Mezzullo, McCandlish and Framme in Richmond, Virginia and author of Virginia's no-fault newborn neurological injury law; Kenneth Niswander, M.D., Professor of Obstetrics and Gynecology at the University of California-Davis in Sacramento; Michael J. Painter, M.D., Associate Professor of Neurology and Pediatrics and Chief of the Division of Child Neurology at the University of Pittsburgh School of Medicine's Children's Hospital in Pennsylvania; and Nigel Paneth, M.D. M.P.H., Associate Professor of Pediatric and Public Health at Columbia University and the G. H. Sergievsky Center in New York City.

Our registration fee was $90, and we limited attendance to the first 150 registrants. We sent a symposium brochure to 30 attorneys, most of whom I knew from my prior depositions or trial testimonies. Members of the Wisconsin Society of Obstetrics and Gynecology received a brochure as did all of the Wisconsin neonatologists. A few brochures were sent to other sponsoring organizations. Assisting me with the mailings, paper work, coffee breaks, overhead transparency changes, and social hour at the end of the day were Janet Sipes, wife of a Green Bay obstetrician, and my wife Crystal - a true Mom and Pop production.

Following my opening remarks and description of the symposium's objectives, the 141 registrants from Wisconsin, Michigan, Minnesota and Illinois welcomed our first speaker, Dr. Niswander. Other speakers followed, and all of them were well informed on their subject matter and gave excellent presentations. Perhaps the highlight of the day was the 45-minute panel discussion with all the speakers answering questions regarding the appropriate and inappropriate testimony relating to the probable cause of CP in the individual patient. I had prepared transparencies of experts' testimony which Janet and Crystal projected, and Dr. Utrie would ask individual panel members to give their opinion on the accuracy or quality of the experts' testimony.

Finally, the formal part of the symposium ended, and the social hour began with the announcement of winners of the quiz that the registrants had completed earlier. At that time, and throughout the 1980s and 1990s, I made a point to distribute a quiz to conference attendees prior to my presentations. We did this as well at this symposium. In this case, seven registrants answered all but one of the questions correctly and had to share the champagne as the prize.

The entire symposium was taped since we had several requests to do so from individuals unable to attend. Dr. Utrie, who had been conducting the Panel portion of the program, made some closing remarks followed by my own ending remarks:

DR. UTRIE: Okay. Thank you. Well, I believe that concludes the cases that Herb has selected. I'd just like to take this opportunity to thank the members of the program committee, and particularly Herb Sandmire. I think that all of you know him. If we didn't have an individual with his energy and dedication and intensity, a program like this never could have been presented, and in particular, the fine faculty which he assembled. I think you really deserve a round of applause, Herb.

DR. SANDMIRE: Well, thank you very much. Before we announce the prize winners, I really want to express my appreciation to the fine speakers. I couldn't believe that I could call these people up on the phone and have them say, sure, I'll come to Oshkosh, Wisconsin. And that really made the program feasible. Obviously, without Dr. Paneth, Dr. Painter, Mr. Grimstad, Ms. Sandy Kramer, Dr. Niswander and Dr. Hack, we wouldn't have had this kind of program. So the ability to put on the program was entirely dependent upon the willingness of these expert professionals within their respective disciplines to share their knowledge and information with us.

On September 22, 1989 I gave an annual address to ACOG District VI Junior Fellows in St. Paul, Minnesota entitled "Exposing the Cerebral Palsy Myth." The following month, on October 11, 1989, I addressed the Northeastern Wisconsin Perinatal Center attendees with a presentation entitled "Modern Concepts of Cerebral Palsy Causation." In addition, I spoke to the Berlin Hospital Association Medical and Nursing staff on July 8, 1991, regarding "Cerebral Palsy is it preventable?" In July of 1991, I gave a similarly titled presentation at the Tenth Annual Community Health Network Summer Conference in conjunction with the Oshkosh Experimental Aircraft Convention.

CHAPTER 33

Legislative forum

A LEGISLATIVE FORUM, in response to high medical liability insurance costs, was organized by my two co-chairpersons, Janet Sipes and Crystal Sandmire, and me,. The title of our forum was "The Medical Liability Crises: A Community Forum." Sponsoring organizations included the Brown County Medical Society and the Coalition for Fairness in Medical Litigation (an organization I had started earlier in the year).

Speakers included representatives from hospitals, the nursing and medical profession, business, labor and the Green Bay Health Department. Nine legislators were also in attendance.

The *Green Bay Press Gazette*, reported on the forum in its December 8, 1987 paper:

> **Medical group calls for legal reform**, By *Terry Anderson*
> *Fearful and frustrated by a legal system that they believe resembles a lottery, a coalition of Wisconsin medical specialists have initiated a drive for legal reform.*
>
> *The Coalition for Fairness in Medical Litigation met Monday evening in the Regency Conference Center. Speakers hammered away at the problems presented by sky-rocketing medical malpractice insurance costs. Nearly 200 people attended the session.*
>
> *Green Bay orthopedic surgeon, David Jones said one out of three orthopedic specialists in Wisconsin has been sued for medical malpractice.*
>
> *The vast majority of the lawsuits have no merit, Jones said, However, because the contingency fee system does not require paying a lawyer unless there is a settlement, there is no reluctance to file suit.*

"The public in general has developed a lottery mentality," he said.

Obstetrician John Utrie said liability insurance for his specialty has increased from about $5,500 to $44,000 during the past six years. "Ultimately, if this continues to go on, we'll have difficulty in the delivery of care."

Utrie said last year the University of Wisconsin Medical School did not produce a single specialist in obstetrics, in large part because of the malpractice crisis.

Green Bay physician Herbert Sandmire, an outspoken advocate for litigation reform, said the coalition was started by the Wisconsin Association of Obstetricians and Gynecologists, the medical specialty that has probably been the hardest hit by the rise in insurance premiums.

Other physician groups have joined the organization which is presenting a 12-point package of reform to the state Legislature, similar to measures already taken in Indiana and California, said Sandmire. Sandmire said the majority of malpractice suits that are filed have no merit.

CHAPTER 34

Eastern European Countries

WE WERE INVITED by Dr. Brooks Ranney and his wife Vi to join them and 36 others on a lecture tour of East Germany, Czechoslovakia, Hungary, Bulgaria, Yugoslavia and Poland from May 23, 1988 to June 11, 1988. Each of these countries, at the time, was under Communist control, although the grip was weakening.

It was interesting to find out that married couples from these countries were not allowed to go abroad together because of the possibility of escaping to a Western country. If physicians came to the United States for attendance at medical meetings, they could not be accompanied by their spouses.

With our hosts in each country, we enjoyed daily meetings filled with presentations of research papers by physicians from each group. I gave a paper entitled "Shoulder dystocia complicating obstetrical delivery" at the William Pick Medical College on the third day of the trip and presented my research entitled "Fertility after IUD discontinuation" at Debrecen Medical College in Debrecen, Hungary and at Warsaw Medical College in Poland during the last week of the trip.

Vi Ranney was a very competent professional tour leader who made our trip relaxing and enjoyable. When we crossed into Czechoslovakia from East Germany, we observed that people can exist under oppressed conditions and still retain a sense of humor, such as when an East German soldier border guard called his buddy over to peruse Crystal's passport and exclaimed in perfect English "**old photo.**" Actually it was an outdated picture even though the passport was up to date.

While in Warsaw we got lost. We had walked over to a huge department store from our hotel. The store seemed to cover two or three blocks with multiple entrances and exits. When we vacated the store, we apparently left by an unintended exit and walked in the wrong direction before finally admitting to ourselves that we were lost. Being quite "astute worldwide travelers," we solved our dilemma by flagging a taxi, giving the driver the name of our hotel and, instantly, we were no longer lost.

The Berlin wall came down about a year after our tour. I have often reflected on how happy the physicians we met probably were with their newfound freedom.

CHAPTER 35

Dr. En-Lan Xia

IN THE FALL of 1988, Dr. En-Lan Xia was sent to the University of Wisconsin Medical School to recruit a visiting professor for the Department of Obstetrics and Gynecology for her medical school in Beijing. Dr. Jan Byrd, her University of Wisconsin Medical School hostess, arranged for her to spend two weeks with me in Green Bay. At the end of those two weeks, she asked me to become the Honored Professor for her medical school.

The October 22, 1988 *Green Bay Press Gazette article by Sean Schultz* described some of her experiences in Green Bay as well as her experiences at the time of the Cultural Revolution, which ended in 1978:

> **Visitor marvels at local hospital**
> **Chinese doctor learns about birth, U.S.-style**
> *Like new parents comparing notes on their children's first steps, Drs. Herbert Sandmire and Xia En-Lan have spent the past two weeks talking babies.*
>
> *Their talks, however, were of a clinical nature. Sandmire, an obstetrician-gynecologist in the Medical Arts Building at 704 S. Webster Ave, was a host to Dr. Xia En-Lan, a visiting fellow from Beijing, China.*
>
> *Sandmire was showing off his "babies" – his practice and the related departments at St. Vincent and Bellin Memorial hospitals.*
>
> *Xia, who came to Green Bay from clinical and hospital observations in Madison, will remain in the United States until February studying gynecological and obstetrical methods.*
>
> *Sandmire hopes to pay her a visit in Beijing in the summer of 1990 as a lecturer and instructor for several weeks. Xia will then*

have the opportunity to put her babies on display. She is head of the ob/gyn department at FuXing Hospital and associate professor at the Capital Institute of Medicine, both in Beijing.

Xia said her visit to the United States came at the invitation of Dr. Janis Byrd, a physician in family practice in Madison and a professor of family medicine at the University of Wisconsin Health Science Center there. Byrd met Xia during a visit to China in 1981.

Sandmire is director of the UW Family Practice Obstetrical Rotation in Green Bay and of the Visiting Fellowship Program for Obstetrics, sponsored by the Continuing Medical Education Department, Health Science Center at Madison.

Xia's trip is both a cultural and educational exchange, one that has come about since China initiated liberal reforms in 1978.

"We import and exchange advanced knowledge and technical skills from foreign countries," she said. "We have gotten a lot of progress, but in the developed countries their progress is improved more quickly."

"In our country doctors are more respected by people because doctors serve the people," said Xia. "Our government says serve the people wholeheartedly."

She practiced medicine at Beijing hospitals until 1970 when she was separated from her husband and two children and sent to Gan-Su Province during the Cultural Revolution.

Sandmire said the move was a punitive one by the Chinese goverment against those with higher educations "who were thought to have too good an opinion of themselves."

But it was punishment with purpose. Xia said, when she arrived in Gan-Su Province, there was an empty field where a hospital was to be. It took 18 months to get a hospital erected, and she and the rest of the medical staff pitched in to help the workers with construction!!!.

She trained three nursing classes each year until she left in 1978. More than 100 nurses and 50 doctors were trained. "After 10 years they are grown up and now the government asked us to come back to Beijing."

Xia said her government has asked the population to carry out family planning, limiting families to just one child.

"Our government hopes our population will control certain numbers so deaths and births make balance," she said.

It isn't working yet because with a higher standard of living, the people are living longer and the birth rate still exceeds the death rate. "Birth control can't catch up," said Xia.

Because most women have just one baby, Xia said 96 percent of the deliveries at her hospital are first-time births. As a result, 20 to 25 percent of the deliveries are done by Caesarean section.

The visiting fellow was intrigued by the video tapes Sandmire has prepared for medical students and resident training purposes. She left with a complete set of ringbooks filled with updated information compiled by Sandmire as well as many of his lecture tapes.

The most impressive characteristic of Dr. Xia was her expression of politeness and her appreciation of what she learned while in Green Bay. These are exemplified in the following letter written by her at the conclusion of her two weeks in Green Bay.

Dr. Sandmire
Ob-Gyn Associates of Green Bay, Ltd.
704 So. Webster Avenue
Green Bay, Wisconsin 54301
Dear Dr. Sandmire,

Thank you indeed for your effort for my study when I was in Green Bay and thank your wife again for her kindly help. I was moved deeply by your friendship, good arrangement, patient teaching and your precious gift – five compilations of update obstetrical materials. I will remember it forever.

Although two weeks is to me too short to learn from you, I still studied a lot. Your operation skill, you work so hard and conscientious[ly], you exert yourself in the obstetrical and gynecological science and technology. You have some creative opinion in obstetrical practice which I heard in your video tapes that I will never forget. You are my respected teacher and friend. I wish that I will have the fortune to study from you again in China in the future.

Sincerely yours,
En-Lan Xia

Her kind words continued in her May 7, 1989 letter:

Dear Dr. Sandmire:

I was so surprised when I received your file mailed from post office. This new information [sic] are needed in our developing country very much. I do like it. I have put it into my five filation already and I will and have read it in detail. Thank you and your dear wife indeed.

Chinese VCR is different from your country's and then the video tape cannot been [sic] showed here. I have sent those tapes to a broadcast station to change it into Chinese style.

Our hospital have [sic] set up a new department recently named Perinatal Medicine Research Center. The Chairmen of our Hospital Mr. De-Xiang Li told me that we would like and hope eagerly to invite you to act as a Honor Professor and an advisor of this center. I don't know if you agree with us? Please let me know. We will send you a letter of appointment.

Since I came back I always missed you and your wife. Your video tape, filation, newspaper and picture are best things for me to remember you and our friendship. I often saw them.

Wish we will meet again in China.

Thank you again

Yours Sincerely, En-Lan Xia

The aftermath of the Tiananmen Square protests of June 4, 1989 hampered U.S. and Chinese cultural and educational exchanges and prevented my 1990 visit to Fu-Xing Hospital. I had been invited to become the Honored Professor and Advisor to the recently formed Perinatal Medicine Research Center. My responsibilities were to travel to their hospital and teach the Chinese Obstetrics for eight weeks every other year. Although my 1990 visit was cancelled by the Chinese government, I continued to send Dr. En-Lan Xia reprint articles as well as video tapes of my more recent lectures, which she adapted to Chinese VCR. It is amazing that citizens of two countries that are unfriendly to each other can have individual citizens expressing their mutual friendship and respect.

CHAPTER 36

South American Adventure

IN THE SPRING of 1989, we went on the South American Adventure, a two-week trip sponsored by the Wisconsin Alumni Association. We visited Peru, Chile, Argentina and Brazil. The trip began in Lima, Peru, where we felt like we'd gone back in time while walking the streets among Inca Indians leading their llamas and peddling their wares - such poverty and such "hawking" to try to get some American money. If they couldn't sell you something, they tried to steal anything they could grab away from you. We really had to be careful. Some members of our group had things taken right from their suitcases as they were being transported from the hotel room to the airport.

During this trip, we visited one of the most amazing and mystical places in the world - Machu Picchu – a large Incan city discovered just 78 years ago after being hidden under jungle growth for four centuries. The city built far up on a mountain in the Andes is intact but for the straw roofs that have long since rotted away. We reached this area on a switch back train. Half way up the mountain, the train had to stop because of a "rock slide" that had recently covered the track. Some suspected that this occurrence was not an accident, but rather damage caused by "the Shining Path guerillas." In fact, while the track was being cleared and repaired, a guerilla came out of the woods and just wandered around the train carrying his gun. We were told to ignore him and to get back on the train, instead of walking around and watching the repair. After hours of repair and delay, we continued to Machu Picchu.

We spent the next day in Lima, Peru's capital, before flying to Buenos Aires, Argentina by way of Santiago, Chile. Buenos Aires, often referred to as the "Paris of South America," is one of the largest cities in the Western Hemisphere. Our Sheraton Hotel was wonderful, the city was clean, the shopping was good, and we felt relatively safe. The ever-present throngs of poverty-stricken Argentinians were on the streets, but they were not as aggressive as those of Peru. One day we were taken to a ranch on the Pampas. We were treated to a real gaucho festival of song, dance and horse shows, with gauchos showing off their skills. We had a huge feast, a chance to swim in their pool, a ride on the horses, and finally a buggy ride.

Brazil was our next destination. We flew directly to Iguassu on Argentina Airlines. All our flights were smooth and uneventful. A bus took us directly to Iguassu Falls on the Argentina side. At one point, crossing the Parada River, we could see Paraguay, Argentina and Brazil all at the same time. If you have seen Niagara Falls and thought it "great," wait until you see Iguassu. The Rio Iguassu widens to a distance of two miles just above the precipice over which the river drops 200 feet to create spectacular falls. Torrents of water fall in dozens of cataracts among the jungle greenery. The most spectacular cataract is Devil's Throat. We walked out on catwalks over the river and to the edge of the falls to take pictures. Of course the best views were from the helicopter ride we were to take later over the falls.

On to customs – first in Argentina, then in Brazil. This should have gone smoothly, except that one man couldn't find his passport. Finally, the bus took the rest of us to the hotel in Brazil and left that couple sitting there at customs until our guide could resolve the problem. We found out later that we had a very rich kleptomaniac in our group – a revelation made possible by her self-admission when later confronted. Apparently kleptomaniacs psychologically obtain a "high" concerning the possibility of being caught that is the motivation for their continued thievery. I do not know if sexual gratification is also achieved, but I never claimed to be a psychiatrist and so have no expertise in the field.

After a great dinner and breakfast the next morning (everywhere we went the breakfasts were great – quite different than on our Eastern European trip), we took a helicopter ride over the falls. Unbelievable – four of us and the pilot. There was a small open window through which we could video the whole thing. This trip was one thrill after another.

We went on a city tour of Rio de Janeiro. It was obvious that Rio had been a magnificent city in the past, but it now showed a lot of neglect. Brazil, and especially Rio, had no money to keep up all the parks, ocean beaches and boulevards with reflecting pools, the latter now filled with debris. Rio used to be the capital before Brasilia was built, and it has since lost some of its importance. The thrilling experience in Rio was the cable car ride to the top of Sugarloaf Mountain (1300 feet tall). This is where a James Bond movie was filmed. The day we went up, we were delayed a bit while equipment for a movie was transported to the top.

We skipped some trips into the mountains and out to the ranches for the next couple days and reflected on the fact that great big Brazil, prior to its independence, was owned by tiny Portugal. I spent a couple of bad days with intestinal problems, eating nothing but chicken broth and trying to get better for the long flight home back to snow.

We enjoyed our trip tremendously, and with the exception of the kleptomaniac, we enjoyed our fellow travelers. Given the repeated bad news we'd read about Peru, Argentina, and Brazil every time we could find an English newspaper (strikes, bad economy, guerilla activity, riots, etc.), we were treated surprisingly well. We had very good hotels, wonderful hospitality, and were shown spectacular sights.

CHAPTER 37

Wedding Anniversaries

1988 (37th)

IN JULY OF 1988, while Sweetie and I were attending the annual meeting of the Wisconsin section of ACOG at the Landmark Resort in Egg Harbor, we were surprised by the arrival of all of our children and their significant others as well as 9-month old grandson Kyle. The significant others were Tony Munda, Ed Zimmer, Beth Weir, and Tracy Kristofferson. The occasion was an early 37th anniversary of our marriage (September 15, 1951).

Amazingly, the planning was without leaks, and we would never have suspected it despite the summertime being the best opportunity for everyone to be free at the same time. It was indeed a very pleasant surprise for Sweetie and me, and the kids enjoyed the social activities of our meeting, especially the traditional Door County evening fish boil. Significant others who did not lead to marriage were Tracy and Ed. Subsequently Dave and Beth married and Cheryl and Tony were divorced.

2001 (50th). Ixtapa trip, November 17-24, 2001.

Our 50th wedding anniversary celebration took place at Club Med in Ixtapa, Mexico with our five children, their five spouses and ten grandchildren. The only one missing was Corky's Hanna. It was all we expected and more. To our surprise, the kids had made a "This is your Life" video about one and one-half hours of pictures, movies and comments by each of our kids. David coordinated it with contributions sent to him by the others. They arranged to have a room there at Club Med, ordered flowers, a cake and champagne, and had a VCR to show the video. Cher and Vonnie coordinated making a neat scrapbook containing a double page made by each of the 21 of them with pictures and comments of their choosing. Both of those gifts are real treasures.

The week starting November 17 (for all except Dave who came late at mid-week because of teaching responsibilities) and ending November 24th, was fun-filled with lots of activities included in the package. There was a baby club where grandchildren Cam and Mac spent some time, giving Lisa and Mike time to do other things. There were at least two other sets of twins – both a little older and running around. I think it was almost easier having Mac and Cam not walking – just crawling a bit – so that they were easier to keep track of. Their brother Andrew spent a little time in the toddler club but mostly enjoyed the pool and beach with the rest of us.

Just walking on the beach and climbing three flights of stairs every time we went from our room to the dining room were Grandpa and Grandma's main activites. Our other pleasures were the pool and just watching the rest of the family in their activities. We went into town one day to read our email and get phone messages from home.

Most of the group went parasailing right off the beach. Alec was the youngest of our group to go. Mostly the Dads and sons did that. Some of us played tennis, while others did archery, basketball, soccer, trampoline, softball and ping-pong. Just before lunch, they had water exercises, followed by pool games for all ages. The pools were so warm that even the babies loved to go swimming in their rings. It was fun to see how all the kids now swam well, and no one was apprehensive about going in.

A new activity none of us had experienced before was trapeze. The first day there, Yvonne took Crystie and Trevor to check out the children's time on the apparatus. Trevor definitely wanted to do it. That surprised no one because he is so active and has little fear of anything. Vonnie went back to her room to get her camera and Beth was busy somewhere else. Vonnie was gone just a few minutes, and when she came back she saw Trevor but not Crystie. She said "Where is Crystie?" Trevor said "Up there." She was just ready to take off. She and Trevor were both six years old at that time. The ladder was a straight-up, metal rung contraption that wiggled as you went up. The platform you took off from, we estimated, was about 35 to 40 feet up. Of course there was a guy there who brought the bar close enough to grab onto with one hand and then catch it with the other as you jumped off. They had a safety strap attached and a big safety net below to fall into. They would swing out, bring their legs up over the bar and swing hanging upside down, then bring their legs back down, do a flip over and come down. Alec did it in the next age group. Of course, the adults did more complicated stuff. Beth, Yvonne, Corky, Cary, Spencer, and Tyler all did it. Yvonne, Corky, Beth and Cary reached the stage where they were caught by a guy on another swinging bar, then letting go, turning, and again catching the bar behind them. It was pretty exciting to watch. Corky and Vonnie were chosen to be in a show put on late in the week, dressed in tights so they looked like real performers. Each night, there was a performance in the open air theatre - musical, comedy or a combination of the two. At the end of the week, they had the kids put on a show. They had been training them in groups during the week.

The grounds were beautiful. Our rooms were near a fenced-in lagoon said to have a crocodile in it. None of us ever saw it, but we did see numerous iguanas (some very large) and an armadillo crawling in the bushes next to the building as well as many beautiful birds. Banana trees were loaded with bunches of bananas.

Three times a day, there was a huge buffet with many, many tables loaded with every kind of food imaginable. It was impossible to try everything, even if you chose something different for each meal. We could eat inside or out and always had three tables close together for our big family.

It was a beautiful vacation enjoyed by everyone and second only to our Alaska cruise in 1998.

CHAPTER 38

Perinatal medicine and the law

DR. WATSON BOWES, JR. began his presentation entitled "Intrapartum fetal monitoring" at the January 1991 meeting of the American Society of Medicine and Law by stating that "the best article appeared a week ago in *Obstetrics and Gynecology* – too late to include in my handout bibliography." "The author," he continued, "who I will ask to stand up to be identified and be available during the break to answer questions." I stood up. Dr. Bowes was an editor for *OB-Gyn Survey* and a recognized national leader in obstetrics.

Several years later, in 2005, I was humbled and flattered to receive a letter from Dr. Bowes relaying to me his change in position on the cause of brachial plexus injury in newborns based, in part, on his review of our studies:

> *Obstetrical and Gynecological Survey*
> *December 30, 2005*
> *Herbert F. Sandmire, MD*
> *Ob-Gyn Associates of Green Bay, Ltd.*
> *704 S. Webster Ave.*
> *Green Bay, WI 54301*
> *Dear Dr. Sandmire;*
> *Thank you for your kind letter of December 12. It was a pleasure and privilege to comment on the obstetrical literature for 13 years in the pages of Survey, and I appreciate knowing that you found the editorials helpful from time to time.*
> *Allow me to return a compliment, if I may. For a number of years I have read with great interest your articles on various topics in clinical obstetrics. I was always impressed that in the midst of a busy*

private practice and without an NIH grant you continued to accomplish meaningful and relevant clinical research. I was especially influenced by your publications about shoulder dystocia and the etiology of brachial plexus injuries. Years ago I was quite convinced that brachial plexus injuries associated with vertex deliveries were in most cases the result of excessive downward traction occurring in the attempt to deliver the anterior shoulder. Regrettably, I even said as much in the chapter I wrote on labor and delivery for the first edition of Maternal-Fetal Medicine *(Creasy and Resnik). Subsequently, it was your article and those of Ray Jennett and later those by Gherman on the subject that convinced me that I should modify my position on that matter, as I did in later editions of the text. I see from the letter by you and Dr. DeMott in the November '05 issue of the Green Journal that you are continuing to educate the obstetrical community on this important subject.*

Best wishes for the New Year.
Sincerely,
Watson A. Bowes Jr., M.D.

During the morning break of the 1991 American Society of Medicine and Law meeting, a lawyer from Melbourne, Australia bent my ear with a case that he was defending relating to alleged failure to monitor the fetus properly during labor. I asked him to send me the medical records and assured him that if I found the care appropriate I would be happy to come to Australia as an expert witness to assist in the defense of the physician and Melbourne's Queen Victoria Medical Centre. I received the medical records as well as the legal complaint indicating that one of the twins allegedly was improperly monitored and deprived of adequate oxygen, leading to cerebral palsy. I felt that the care was appropriate, and therefore on September 3, 1991 we checked into the Auckland, New Zealand Travel Lodge en route to Melbourne. That evening, Jennifer Wilson M.D., who I had met at a previous meeting, picked us up at our hotel for a reception at her home. She had also invited her colleagues from her "contraceptive choice" group.

The following day we visited a World War II museum and other sights prior to our flight to New Zealand's South Island. At a stopover in Christ Church, we heard over the intercom that a physician was needed to attend to an arriving passenger. I said to Sweetie, "I hope it's a woman about to have a baby." It wasn't. It happened to be a middle-aged man, pale, cold, clammy and perspiring with a heart rate of 40. It was an obvious vasovagal response causing a slow heart rate, perhaps because of fear. In his response to my questioning, the passenger reported no previous heart or respiratory problems. With this information I was able to reassure him, after which he made a remarkable improvement presumably due to less anxiety. I advised the airline captain and the flight attendant to call for an ambulance to take him to a hospital for further evaluation.

Even though it was not a woman about to have a baby, the captain and co-captain were pleased with my "pretending to be an internist" and invited me to ride shot gun (immediately behind them) for the remainder of the flight to Queenstown in the South Island. The view was great for our video camera.

While in Queenstown, we took a bus trip to beautiful Milford Sound. Another day we took a cable car up 446 meters to the Skyland Restaurant on top of Bob's Peak where we enjoyed a good dinner. Next we arrived at a beautiful hotel in Melbourne. While there, we took a bus tour to watch the Penguin Parade as they came out of the ocean at dusk.

I never did get on the witness stand in the legal case since the "life-expectancy" expert decreased his life expectancy opinion markedly and the case was settled.

We left Melbourne and headed for tropical Cairns in northern Australia nearer the equator. While there we saw pictures of the old Pacific Hotel where my brother-in-law Theron had spent some time during World War II. We took a trip out to the Great Barrier Reef, a spectacular sight indeed. While there we boarded a mini-submarine to view the coral – not enjoyable for me because of my severe claustrophobia.

Our 40th wedding anniversary was coming up on September 15, 1991, and we did not know if we should celebrate it on the September 15th Green Bay date or the September 15th Cairns date. We decided to celebrate both dates to make sure the anniversary of our marriage was properly enjoyed.

I have begun this segment with Dr. Bowes commenting on my article, "Whither Electronic Fetal Monitoring (EFM)," as well as my other research articles, and will close with an unsolicited letter from Mayo Clinic gynecologist, Raymond A. Lee, M.D., who also commented on the above article and my opinion that EFM was introduced into general use prior to its proven benefit.

Mayo Clinic
Rochester, Minnesota 55905
Raymond A. Lee, M.D.
Gynecologic Surgery
December 12, 1990
Herbert F. Sandmire, M.D.
704 South Webster Avenue
Green Bay, WI 54301
Dear Doctor Sandmire:

I rarely have written to an author of any medical journal other than to inquire or ask a question about the content of the article which most frequently was an area of interest to me.

I am writing to you now regarding your clinical commentary on fetal monitoring. I am out of obstetrics but was interested more from the perspective of the potential benefits of the new technologies with which we are all working. I am suspicious that the new technologies of urodynamics in evaluating the incontinent patient fall into the same category as fetal monitoring. I do not have a randomized, prospective study, but I have almost on a daily basis clinical evidence that would suggest there is gross overutilization, confusion, and conflicting data for urodynamics, etc.

However, that is not the point of your manuscript; and I just wish to compliment you on undertaking this endeavor and the very effective way you have carried out the discussion. I think it's another example of the need to critically analyze "new advances." I am not unaware that what appears to be a radical departure in one generation can be accepted as the most conservative treatment by the next generation. It is only that I would hope these new advances are, in fact, not a step backwards in the care of our patients.

Again, congratulations on your fine manuscript.
Sincerely,
Raymond A. Lee, M.D

CHAPTER 39

Teaching fly-in physicians

THE FAMOUS EXPERIMENTAL Aircraft Association head-
quartered in Oshkosh, Wisconsin, sponsors an annual weeklong fly-in
late in July. In conjunction with the fly-in, the Berlin Memorial Hospital through its Community Health Network sponsors a medical conference for fly-in physicians. The medical conferences began in 1980
and continue to the present time. I was an invited speaker for the first
time in 1992. Most speakers were required to fill a two-hour time slot
for which we received $750.00.

The meeting was always held at the beautiful Heidel House Resort
in Green Lake, Wisconsin, 25 miles west of Oshkosh. The speakers and
their spouses were all invited to a pre-meeting dinner at a fancy, lake-
side restaurant each Thursday evening. The meeting took place on Friday and Saturday morning. Friday evening we were all treated to the
sponsors' famous steak-fry.

The combination of recreation and the participation in the continuing medical education for fly-in physicians from all across the United
States was especially rewarding and gratifying. The appreciation
expressed by the audience physicians, as reflected in their speaker evaluation forms was helpful in knowing we were usually "on the right
tract" in what we were presenting.

I participated in seven consecutive annual conferences. The content
of one of my two hours was typically an update about what was new in
obstetrics and gynecology. Titles for the other hour included "Cerebral
Palsy: Is it preventable?", "Gyn Oncology," "Does the large fetus cause
large problems?", "Labor management – pitfalls to avoid," "The diagnosis and treatment of cervical intraepithelial neoplasia: when to look
and when to LEEP," "Legal issues in medicine with the presentation of

a mock (based on an actual trial) trial," and in 1994, "Obstetrics for the 1990s – return to the 1960s."

At the beginning of this last lecture, I pointed out the advances which had occurred since the 1960s: The development of neonatal intensive care units was by far the most important, followed by prevention of Rh-related problems, prevention of the rubella newborn syndrome by vaccination, ability to diagnose Down's syndrome and other genetic abnormalities early in pregnancy, and the prevention of newborn hepatitis by the vaccination of young women. Also important was the three-fold reduction in neural tube defects (spina bifida and anencephaly) by prescribing 0.4 milligrams of folic acid daily before and during each pregnancy.

In that "Return to the 1960s" lecture, I pointed out that change in the way we, as obstetricians, do things does not necessarily result in better cost-effective care. I cited as examples electronic fetal monitoring, over-use of epidurally-administered medication for labor pain relief, a five-fold increase in cesarean deliveries, routine cesarean for breech presenting fetuses, over use of ultrasound, the cerebral palsy causation myth, over-emphasis on the Friedman labor curve, external version during delivery of twin B, low-dose pitocin utilization, and over-reliance on ultrasonic estimates of fetal weight.

An analysis of the feedback provided by some of the comments on the speaker evaluation forms demonstrates this one-hour lecture to be the best and the most appreciated of all of my 14 hours of presentations to this group:

> *Probably the most enlightening speech on OB I've heard in my career.*
> *Fantastic talk – as usual.*
> *Great update and review. Fantastic.*
> *Superb argument and presentation.*
> *Valuable.*
> *Always outstanding.*
> *Always good.*
> *Excellent.*

As can be seen from comments on the evaluation forms the physician audience changed very little from year to year. The evaluation forms were mailed to me by Elliot Goldin, MD, Director, CME Committee, along with the following letter:

Community Health Network

August 24, 1994
Dear Herb:
Again, thank you for your participation in our 14th Annual BMH Summer Conference held on July 28, 29 & 30, 1994 at the Heidel House Resort & Conference Center in Green Lake.

Enclosed please find a check for your honorarium. As always, the participants enjoyed your presentations. It was nice that you and your wife were again able to be part of our program and hope you had a safe trip home.

If you have any questions or concerns, please feel free to contact me.

Sincerely, Elliot G. Goldin MD

Handwritten note at the bottom of the letter by Elliot: Everyone had very positive remarks on your talks, Herb. Thanks very much. Elliot

The speakers were also largely the same year after year which led to friendships, one of which was with William R. Jewell MD, Chief of General, Thoracic and Oncologic Surgery at Kansas University. He sent me a nice letter following the 1994 meeting:

Kansas University Surgery Association
Kansas City, Kansas 66160-7308

August 8, 1994
Dear Herb,
Thank you for sending the videotape and the other information. I have a feeling that some of our faculty people in OB/GYN could use this information. I really enjoyed your talk last Saturday morning.

I hope we will all get together again up there. I have been impressed with the attendees as well as the speakers. Sheila and I are looking forward to seeing you and Crystal and all of the others in a year.

Kind Regards, William R. Jewell, M.D. Chief of Section

One Saturday morning at 7:45 am, I received a call in my room 15 minutes before I was to begin my two hours of lectures informing me that a one-hour speaker was involved in an auto accident driving from Chicago and would be unavailable for the meeting. "Could I fill in for one hour for the absent speaker?" Having nothing prepared I said I would suggest a one-hour question-and-answer session. If they didn't like that idea or didn't have sufficient questions, I threatened them by saying I would deliver a one-hour monologue. Toward the end of my session, with the questions seeming to be coming less frequently, I dragged out my answers and sounded like a tape recorder with a weak battery.

My honorarium, as a result of my extra hour, was increased from $750 to $1000.

CHAPTER 40

Cesarean consultant

WHILE ATTENDING THE CAOG meeting in October of 1993, Dr. Alfred Kobak of Valparaiso, Indiana asked me to be a cesarean consultant for their Porter   Memorial Hospital. He repeated this request in this November 1993 letter:

> *Porter Memorial Hospital*
> *814 LaPorte Avenue*
> *Valparaiso, Indiana 46383*
> *November 22, 1993*
> *Herbert F. Sandmire, M.D.*
> *704 South Webster*
> *Green Bay, Wisconsin 54301*
> *Dear Herb,*
> *I enjoyed our conversation at the Central Association meeting. I look forward to you visiting Porter Memorial Hospital to help us obtain a better understanding of how our c-section rate can be reduced. Would you please supply us with some dates that are most convenient for you? We plan to have our statistics to you three to four weeks in advance of the scheduled date for your visit. If you have any further requests of us, please do not hesitate to call. Thank you.*
> *Very truly yours,*
> *Alfred Kobak, M.D.*
> *Chief, Department of Obstetrics*

He (Dr. Kobak) had been aware of our first two cesarean papers presented at CAOG meetings and subsequently published in the *JAOG*. The titles of these were "The Green Bay cesarean study I: the physician factor as a determinant of cesarean birth rates" and "The Green Bay cesarean birth study II: The physician factor as a determinant of cesarean birth rates for failed labor."

After receiving his statistics, I analyzed each of the 13 obstetrician's prior total cesarean rates as well as their rates by indication for non-progressive labor, fetal intolerance of labor, repeat cesareans, breech position, and all other causes.

Initially, to implement the goal of reducing the rate of cesarean deliveries, I provided a two-hour lecture on February 10, 1994 to Northwestern Indiana physicians entitled "Identifying determinants of cesarean birth rates." The objective of my lecture was to "provide a discussion of the current factors in obstetrical care that influence route-of-delivery decisions and the effect of the delivery route on maternal and newborn outcomes."

Following this lecture, I met with the Porter Memorial Hospital obstetric nurses to advise them of nursing strategies that may decrease patient requests for a cesarean birth.

I then met individually with each of the 13 obstetricians to discuss their total individual cesarean rates and cesarean rates for each indication. We then discussed how their rates might be decreased while still maintaining optimal outcomes for both mother and baby. The whole process used the same method as that of our first two Green Bay cesarean birth papers although we did not have individual discussions with Green Bay obstetricians. In all, my role as a cesarean birth consultant involved three flights to Chicago where we were met by a limousine for the 75-mile trip to Valparaiso.

On one of those trips to Valparaiso, we made a video entitled "Grandma Crys goes to Valparaiso," especially for our grandson Alec, who at age three worshipped "limos." We filmed her in her best business suit, getting into the "limo" at O'Hare, during the travel while she was napping, and exiting the "limo,"in Valparaiso and did the same for the return trip. Alec cherished the video and hoped he could sometime in his life ride in a "limo."

Following my two-hour February 10, 1994 lecture, we received a letter of appreciation from Dr. Kobak on February 28, 1994:

Porter Memorial Hospital
814 LaPorte Avenue
Valparaiso, Indiana 46383
February 28, 1994
Herbert F. Sandmire, M.D.
OB-GYN Associates of Green Bay, LTD.

704 S. Webster Avenue
Green Bay, Wisconsin 54301
Dear Herb:
I greatly appreciated the time you spent at Porter Memorial Hospital, sharing your knowledge and experiences. We hope that this will be helpful in effecting change. The studies and information you have completed are most beneficial to OB/GYN practices outside of the metropolitan teaching centers.
Attached are the results of the evaluation forms returned.
Very truly,
Alfred Kobak, M.D.
Chief, Department of Obstetrics

Another letter of May 10, 1994 from Dr. Kobak further discussed the work in progress toward their goal of reducing cesarean rates while preserving optimal maternal and newborn outcomes.

Porter Memorial Hospital
814 LaPorte Avenue
Valparaiso, Indiana 46383
May 10, 1994
Herbert Sandmire, M.D.
OB-GYN Associates of Green Bay, LTD.
704 S. Webster Avenue
Green Bay, WI 54301
Dear Dr. Sandmire:
Thank you for your March 3 and March 19, 1994 letters. We initiated the non-progressive labor and induction study data collection March 1, 1994. Plans are to accumulate this data for a 4-6 month period and stratify it as you suggested. At the March 1994 OB-GYN Department meeting, a summary of your presentation was reviewed with the focus to support each obstetrician's efforts to reduce their c-section rate. We would be glad to share our additional data with you when it is completed, which should be in early fall 1994.
We appreciate you providing us with the well-organized periodical resource manuals. We have informed the obstetricians and family practitioners of their availability.
Again, thank you for your assistance in our c-section performance improvement project and your continued interest.
Yours truly,
Alfred Kobak, M.D.
Chief, OB/GYN Department

During the early 1990s, with cesarean rates escalating, the print media began to draw attention to the variation in cesarean rates for individual obstetricians and hospitals. Excerpts from the Gary, Indiana September 18, 1994 *Post-Tribune* indicated that "NWI (northwest Indiana) has the most c-sections in Indiana." The article further reported that:

> *Lake and Porter counties average is more than twice Fort Wayne's; doctors and hospitals struggle with cutting back.*
>
> *Northwest Indiana boasts the highest average rate of Cesarean section deliveries in the state of Indiana. The average rate for eight Lake and Porter county hospitals delivering babies is 28.8 percent, more than double Fort Wayne's rate of 13.6 percent, nearly twice Lafayette's 15 percent and higher than South Bend (17.76), Kokoma (26.3) and Indianapolis (22.35). Area doctors and hospital administrators cite several reasons, including a fear of litigation, physician convenience, past practice and financial rewards.*
>
> *Indiana has two malpractice premium rates: for Lake County and the rest of the state. Malpractice insurers point to the area's proximity to Chicago and the high number of lawsuits filed against Northwest Indiana doctors as contributing to an environment of defensive medicine. Obstetricians are among the most frequently sued physicians.*
>
> *The problem of Caesarean section or C-section deliveries is not just local. U.S. rates for C-sections, the most frequently performed surgical operation in the country, are higher than any major industrial nation.*
>
> *The medical consumers' organization, Public Citizen's Health Research Group, stated in its 1994 report, "Unnecessary Caesarean Sections: Curing A National Epidemic," that 473,000 of the nation' 966,000 Caesareans performed in 1992 were unnecessary.*
>
> *"Those Caesareans cost $1.3 billion in unnecessary health expenditures. Almost 40 million Americans have health insurance," said Mary Gabay, a staff researcher and co-author of the Public Citizen Caesarean report. "We don't need to spend that money on unnecessary surgery."*
>
> *Gabay said that although the risk of mothers or babies dying during a C-section delivery is low, it's still two to four times greater than for natural childbirth.*
>
> *Repeat Caesareans make up more than one-third of all such operations. One of the reasons Northwest Indiana's rates are so high is the area's relatively low rate of Vaginal Birth after Caesarean (VBAC).*

For years doctors were weaned in their obstetric residency programs on the old medical adage, "Once a Caesarean, always a Caesarean."

But for more than a decade the American College of Obstetrics and Gynecology has advocated VBACs.

Caesarean deliveries also are more expensive, costing from two to three times as much as a natural vaginal delivery. The average cost of a Caesarean delivery in Indiana in the second quarter of 1993 was $4500, compared to the average cost of an uncomplicated natural delivery of $2500. With complications, the costs for both deliveries can double.

Dr. Jack Foltz, a Crown Point obstetrician and the chairman of obstetrics quality assurance at St. Anthony Medical Center in Crown Point said it also helps when hospitals maintain statistics on Caesareans and VBACs.

That's one tool that has been used successfully at Porter Memorial Hospital, whose 1994 C-section rate was 24 percent. D. Alfred Kobak, chairman of the hospital's obstetric department, said Porter Memorial's rate declined to 18.28 during the first six months of 1994 and should end the year at less than 20 percent.

"We hope it will be around 17 percent," said Kobak.

The reduction is not coincidental.

"We recognized that a Caesarean rate in the high-20s was higher than it should be," Kobak said. "We were persuaded that there were simple and effective ways of reducing that rate."

Kobak said the hospital brought in renowned Green Bay, Wis. Obstetrician and author Dr. Herbert Sandmire, who has lectured extensively on Caesarean rate reduction, to work with physicians and staff.

"And we learned that the difference between one hospital's C-section rate and another's was physician attitude and how a physician manages labor," he said.

Kobak said that low C-section rates are going to be benchmarks of quality obstetrics, something by which every hospital and physician will be judged.

On October 25, 1995, I led a discussion at Porter Memorial Hospital regarding identifying determinants of cesarean birth rates and the following day discussed and updated the management of the labor protocol. On June 19, 1996, I gave a lecture to Hobart, Indiana St. Mary's Hospital medical staff entitled "Cesarean birth rates: how to reduce them."

As indicated in the September 18, 1994 *Post-Tribune* newspaper article, Dr. Kobak was happy with their reduction rates beginning in the first six months of 1994. As for myself, I was pleased with the results and humbled by being asked to assist the obstetricians in northwest Indiana.

CHAPTER 41

No more babies

AS AN OBSTETRICIAN, I have had the good fortune to be working in the happiest of the major medical specialties. For 44 years I have had the privilege of sharing the happiness with the parents of newborns, but on September 19, 1996, at age 67, I delivered my last baby. Suddenly and abruptly, I began to sleep all night every night, including weekends, holidays and my birthdays. Over the 44-year period, I delivered an average of 250 babies per year, which was an average number for obstetricians during that time period. The total number was more than 10,000.

My decision to stop delivering babies was reported in two articles by Sean Schultz appearing on September, 20, 1996 in the *Green Bay Press Gazette*. Her articles were comprehensive, well written, and remarkably accurate for covering a span of 44 years. These articles were picked up by the Associated Press and appeared in the Rockford, Illinois *Register Star* on October 14, 1996 - which may have been a "slow news day" in that city:

> **Sandmire's last baby:**
> **Controversial doctor delivered 10,000 children**
> *If you want a delivery, call Pizza Hut. Don't call Dr. Herbert Sandmire.*
>
> *Sandmire, 67, a gynecologist/obstetrician in Green Bay since July 1, 1959, announced Thursday he is closing the window on the obstetric side of his practice.*
>
> *He delivered his last baby Thursday afternoon.*
>
> *But he's leaving doors open marked "gynecologist," "teacher," "expert witness," "researcher" and "pro-choice proponent." Even though the last label has made his east side clinic the target of frequent protests.*

247

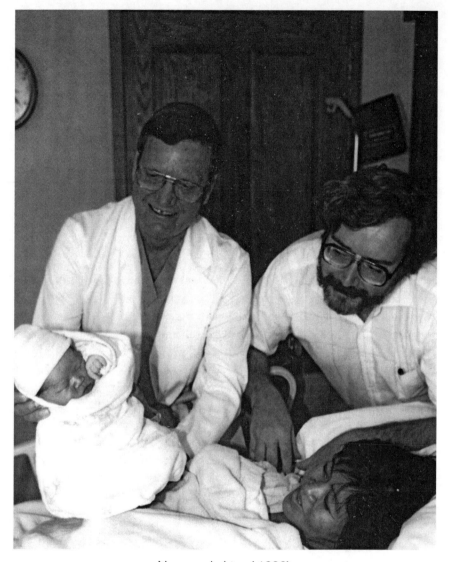

No more babies (1996)

After presiding at the births of more than 10,000 babies since 1953 – more than 9,000 of them in Green Bay – Sandmire has decided he wants to get some sleep at night. Every night. And weekends.

There will be no more late night calls, but fond memories of his scores of patients and their newborns remain.

He can tell you that his first delivery in Green Bay was a boy, Tom Matuszak, the fifth child born to Jackie and Herbert Matuszak.

Jackie stopped having babies after eight. Now she sees Sandmire's son Kevin, an internist, for most of her medical needs.

Sandmire's last delivery was the 8 pound baby girl born to Ray and Dulce Hutchison at 2:17 p.m. Thursday. The baby, the couple's third daughter, wasn't named as of today.

Dulce, surprised to hear she was the last mother to use Sandmire's skills, said it was an honor to be among his patients but "just real surprising" to hear he would give up that part of his work.

"I don't know," she said. "This may be my last one, too."

Sandmire's decision to stop delivering babies caught Sandy Hillman by surprise. The director of the Genesis Center at St. Vincent Hospital where baby Hutchison was born said she's worked with Sandmire for 27 years.

"I learned a lot from him and I'm grateful for that," Hillman said.

Sandmire has seen medicine change in many ways since he began his career as a medical student in 1950, but not much change in babies.

"I have to say they come out about the same way they did in 1950," he teased.

Sandmire admits that he nearly fumbled his first official delivery. But under the circumstances, who could blame him?

It was New Year's Day 1953, and he was a senior medical student called to deliver a baby at a home in Chicago's inner city.

The Rose Bowl was on, and Wisconsin was making a rare appearance. Alan "The Horse" Ameche was running toward the goal line as Sandmire was delivering his first baby. The combination was too much for him. He called the Chicago Maternity Center to report on the delivery and in his excitement, reported that the baby was a boy. She wasn't.

Sandmire has gone on to instruct several hundred other young residents, serving as a full clinical professor in obstetrics, gynecology and family practice medicine with the University of Wisconsin Medical School.

He has lectured in Eastern Europe and presented a host of papers in his field. In the past four months, Sandmire has testified as an expert witness in four medical malpractice cases. He's gone as far as Melbourne, Australia to give testimony.

Since abortion was legalized in 1973, Sandmire has been criticized by abortion opponents for his pro-choice stance.

"My views are pretty typical of obstetricians across the country and even in Green Bay," he said.

Sandmire said if he "withheld certain services from women because it might bring adverse publicity to myself and if women had the legal right for that service.... I would see myself functioning as a barrier to the patient seeking what she had a legal right to have."

He and his wife Crystal raised their five children in Allouez. He's proud of each of them – two of them physicians, along with a gymnastics coach, a photographer and an attorney.

Sandmire gave up his car in 1973 when his environment concerns dictated that he ride a bicycle to work. Even when the temperature was 20 below zero.

For the past 23 years he has given up the comfort of his own bed on those nights when he drew on-call duty. He slept in his office instead, next door to Bellin and St. Vincent hospitals.

Sandmire's original partner, Dr. Stephen Austin, died several years ago. His partners today at OB/GYN Associates include Drs. Richard Bechtel, Robert Cavanaugh and Robert DeMott.

The doctor will still be "in" at his offices in the Medical Arts Building, 704 South Webster Avenue.

He will simply be pursuing his gynecology practice, research, teaching and testimony at a more leisurely pace in daylight.

Doctor's no stranger to controversy

In his 37 years as a gynecologist and obstetrician in Green Bay, Dr. Herbert Sandmire has fit equally well into the roles of kindly family practitioner and fearless women's rights advocate.

He has taken on Green Bay's hospitals and fellow physicians, urging them to lower costs for medical care.

He has taken up the abortion issue, too, challenging those who advocate anti-abortion sentiments with his conviction that women have the right to terminate unwanted pregnancies.

Sandmire didn't sit out the Roe vs. Wade *debate after abortion became legal in 1973. His outspoken support for a woman's right to choose abortion has brought picketers marching outside his offices and occasional acts of vandalism.*

A neighbor, the wife of another doctor, predicted in 1973 that Sandmire's five children would starve because of his defense of women who choose abortion. They didn't.

"It turned out it didn't have any adverse affect on my financial goals, but I was willing to accept that if it did happen," he said.

"If I were an internist, I'd be non-controversial. The issue would be irrelevant to me." Sandmire said.

"I'm not an internist, I'm a gynecologist/obstetrician and in this country the law says women have the right to safe abortions. Why would I say, "No, I'm sorry, I can't help you"?

I'm an advocate for women's health and I'm also able to recognize that some women who have the need for gynecological services will have different philosophies and views than my own" he said. "My own philosophies and views are not important when it comes to providing the best service I can."

On medical advances and reverses: *Sandmire has seen advances in obstetric care but he knows what's gone wrong, too.*

He points to the advancement in "the ability to take care of very tiny babies." But he complains about unnecessarily high Caesarean section rates.

In Green Bay, he's proud to say, the C-section rate is just 10 percent. But why is it 23 percent nationwide?

"Advances have to be truly beneficial to be applauded," Sandmire said.

On managed care: *Sandmire views recent efforts at managed care with misgivings. He said such efforts really aren't new to Green Bay. He and other physicians who opened the Green Bay Surgical Center in 1978 as a low-cost alternative to the hospital setting were ahead of their time.*

To this day, I still miss seeing the happiness expressed by parents at the birth of their baby.

CHAPTER 42

Alaska cruise - Northbound, June 22 - July 4 1998

IN THE SUMMER of 1998, our whole family enjoyed a cruise from Vancouver to Anchorage by way of the Inner Passage along the Canadian coastline. The cruise stops were in Ketchikan, Juneau, Skagway, Haines, Glacier Bay, College Fjords, Seward and finally Anchorage. The calving of the glaciers was an interesting and spectacular sight to witness. Our ship got quite close to this activity. Although beautiful to see, it reminded us that it was a sign of global warming. We saw a village as we went out to a glacier by land, and we were told that the village had not been there just a few years earlier since that area was covered by the glacier.

After a couple days in Anchorage, we traveled by train to Fairbanks with a stopover in Denali Park. The train was great, the scenery was spectacular and the food outstanding. I think it was the first train ride for some of the grandchildren and was quite a thrill for them. Alec, who was five, was really interested in trains, so he was especially excited. Crystie and Trevor were two and one half years old at the time but certainly not too young to enjoy themselves. They got a lot of attention on the ship, especially by the waiters at dinner time. Our waiter would carry them around on his shoulders and even took Trevor into the kitchen to meet the cooks.

For the older grandchildren, I had a daily dollar question. Correct answers would make them one dollar richer. Some questions were of the educational nature. For instance, "What is your cabin number" or "On what deck is your cabin located?" This might come in handy for the younger ones if they got lost on this huge ship. One question I recall was, what color was our Anchorage hotel (it was a dark yellow-brown)? There was no pay out that day as I called the color "shit-brindle," a term few of them had even heard of. Grandma Crys doubted the wisdom of teaching the grandchildren grown-up words! Other questions were – "What is the capital of Alaska?" and "What is the definition of seriatim?"

In Fairbanks we visited what was formerly the 5001st U S Air Force Hospital – now Fort Wainright Hospital, where I was on the OB staff from 1954 to 1956. We enjoyed chatting with the OB nurses who were pleased to obtain the history of my serving as chairperson of the OB department 42 years earlier. Yvonne, having been born in that hospital on January 11, 1956, got on the bed in the room where Sweetie had labored. She posed with her thumb in her mouth, along with her mother, for a photo. One block from the hospital was the apartment (base housing) where we lived for two years. Surprisingly, everything remained as we remembered it 42 years earlier when we rotated home at the conclusion of my Air Force experience. The very same swing set and slide that Cheryl used to play on was outside the back door of the apartment. Obviously it was a very heavy, sturdy metal set which will probably last forever.

While in Fairbanks, at the end of our Princess Cruise, we went on a tour of a gold panning site which provided considerable excitement for the grandchildren who hoping to strike it rich while they swirled the water around in their pans.

There were so many highlights on this trip – the beautiful scenery along the coast up the Inner Passage, the deluxe train trip from Anchorage to Fairbanks through Denali, the sight of Mount McKinley (or Denali, as the natives know it), and just walking the streets of the towns we visited on the way. Revisiting Fairbanks brought back fond memories of my tour of duty 40 years earlier. All of the kids (even Cheryl at the age of 44 but still a kid) had a fabulous time. As I look back on it, I believe it was the best family vacation we ever had.

CHAPTER 43

The "Iron Man who Wasn't (Stroke)

OVER THE YEARS, I had always enjoyed good health and often boasted about never missing a day of work because of illness. As you will see that all changed on May 18, 1999. On May 17, Sweetie and I were returning from Cheboygan, Michigan where I had delivered a lecture to their hospital staff at a breakfast meeting entitled "Safely reducing cesarean rates." It was a nice sunny day for a drive, allowing us to have lunch at our favorite "Log Cabin Restaurant" just north of Escanaba, Michigan. The rest of the drive home was uneventful as was that evening. I slept until 5:30 AM. I showered, shaved and dressed for work. Just as I was attempting to get into my leather jacket to ride my bike to work, I became dizzy, sat down on the chair at the computer, and fell off, awakening Sweetie, who promptly came to where I was in our home office. She called Kevin, who came over quickly, and they took me to St. Vincent Hospital emergency room. They asked me to sign some papers at admittance, and I could not hold the pen. By the time they got me upstairs on a gurney, I could talk and move all four extremities. I even got off the gurney to go to the bathroom.

A carotid artery ultrasound revealed near total blockage of my left internal carotid artery in the neck. Opening my carotid artery was recommended to which I agreed with alacrity. Because I had recovered all of my functions in less than 24 hours, my diagnosis was transient ischemic attack (TIA). By 2 PM that day I was in surgery. It did seem strange, following 46 years of medical practice, to now be a patient and dependent on those fine physicians.

At 5 AM the day following my surgery I experienced a full-blown stroke which rendered me speechless and unable to have a full range of motion with my right hand and arm. They called Sweetie, who got to the hospital within a few minutes. Fortunately, all of my morbidities were temporary, with both my right arm weakness and ability to speak returning over the next seven days.

The only good result of the stroke was being able to see all of our kids and grandkids, all of whom came seriatim (dollar question on the Alaska cruise). Sweetie had alerted all of them about the stroke, saying that she did not think my life was in immediate danger and they did not need to travel home unless they wanted to. When they called to talk to me on the phone, my wife had told them only to ask questions to which I could simply answer yes or no, since my speech was impaired.

After I fully recovered, it has been said that some of my children had speculated on whether my lack of speaking ability would be a good or bad thing!!

The whole experience made me a better doctor and especially more appreciative of Sweetie and all she had done for me over the previous 48 years. I dreaded that she may have to push me around in a wheel chair for the next 20 years, knowing full well that she would willingly do just that. How lucky I am.

As I write this chapter, almost 12 years later, I feel lucky to have had a complete recovery and the ability to accomplish the things I have during that time period.

CHAPTER 44

9/11

ON A PLEASANT Sunday morning, the ninth of September, 2001, we were driving to Baltimore where I was to give testimony in the *Kinner v. Esposito* trial. My testimony was scheduled for Friday morning, the fourteenth of September. The day before we left, we had emailed our children and siblings, alerting them to the possibility of our stopping in Washington D.C. for sight-seeing on the way to Baltimore.

As our trip from Wisconsin went well, we had time to go to the nation's capitol for some sightseeing. Because of the nature of these trials, we were not sure we would be going until the last minute. We did not have a hotel reservation in Washington D.C. and decided to drive to the Washington Mall and take our chances. It was not easy, and after looking for a few hotels on the map without any luck, we happened upon the Crowne Plaza. We stopped and the doorman asked if he could help us. He went in to find out if they had a room. There were only a few left and he said "the least expensive one was $249." (Our kids appreciate this as they really think we need a new car). We think the doorman looked at our car with the duct-taped, damaged back bumper and decided we certainly would not go for an expensive room. But we were glad to get a room at any price, close to everything in town. We did not have enough time to come in from the outskirts each day to see the city.

That afternoon we saw quite a bit of the Smithsonian, had a nice sandwich in the dining room at the Museum of American History, went back to our hotel for a rest, thinking we would do more sightseeing the next morning. There was so much to see. We joked about calling our former governor, Tommy Thompson, now the Secretary Health and Human Services, or our Congressman Mark Green to see if we could

256

get a pass to the Capitol or the White House, but we knew we should have done that well in advance.

When we woke up on 9/11/01, we did not turn on the TV, going down for breakfast instead. When we left the dining room, we noticed a lot of people watching TV in the lobby. We stopped long enough to hear that a plane had hit the World Trade Center in New York. Thinking it was just a bad accident, we went on our way, walking around the park in front of our hotel and then heading toward the White House. From there we were going to walk past the Washington Monument and on to the Capitol. Our hotel was just a few blocks from the White House.

It seemed like we were hearing more sirens than usual, and we commented that there seemed to be people just standing outside buildings – not at bus stops as usual. More fire trucks and police cars passed us and stopped a few blocks ahead. Our curiosity got the best of us so we asked a lady on the street if she knew what was going on. She had heard that a plane had hit the Pentagon and told us the White House was cordoned off and we would not be able to walk in that direction. When we looked like we were having a hard time believing the plane had hit the Pentagon she said, "Well, just look over there, you can see the smoke from it across the river." We decided to walk toward the Smithsonian instead. The street got more and more hectic with emergency vehicles and we found the Smithsonian was also closed.

We headed back to the hotel walking past the Ronald Reagan Building, which is an International Trade Center. There were lots of police around this building, and only daycare parents were allowed to go in to pick up their children. We heard it may be a target, being a trade center. By now, all federal buildings were being evacuated, and the street was gridlocked like we have never seen. Even emergency vehicles could not get through. Cars were lined up trying to get out of underground parking areas. At one point a policeman on a motorcycle came right up on the sidewalk next to us and rode down through people on a crowded sidewalk. How he avoided them was more than we could comprehend. It seemed that everyone was on a cell phone and frustrated when they had trouble getting through.

Along the way we heard that the second Tower in New York had been hit, and it clearly was not an accident. We quickly went to our room, packed our bags as we had to check out by noon. A barrage of emails came to us before we checked out of the Crowne Plaza, including those from our five children at the following times (all Central Daylight):

Vonnie – 8:54 AM
Dave -   9:17 AM
Mike -   9:18 AM

Cheryl -   9:22 AM
Kevin -   10:18 AM

We also had emails from my office people and many friends and relatives, including the Van der Aas from Belgium and the Lammerts-mas from Holland. They all wanted to know where we were and if we were in danger.

We took the time to send an email to each of our kids before we packed up the computer. We knew they would be worried. By the time the hotel personnel were able to get our car out of the garage, traffic was moving on one side of the hotel. Luckily we were headed north (away from the Pentagon) and we could slowly head to Baltimore. Our route took us past the Howard University Hospital, so of course ambulances passed us constantly. As we left the hotel we heard a plane up above us, bringing shivers to us as that is a no fly zone and we were very tense at this point. It turned out to be a fighter jet patrolling the area.

We couldn't get all the victims' families out of our minds, and we were sure it was the same for everyone else. The sun did come up the next morning, and life did go on, but those events left indelible images in our minds. We were again reminded to do our very best each day and appreciate every moment.

Our hotel in Baltimore was in the inner harbor area where all tourist and business activities were closed down because of the 9/11 tragedy. None of the boat tours were available. The only business open, for which we were thankful, was Hooters, an establishment we had not previously patronized, but we got our meals there. For the next two days we spent our time going on long walks, watching TV and preparing for my trial testimony.

The trial was only slightly behind schedule despite being closed Tuesday afternoon on 9/11. I was on the witness stand all afternoon Friday, September fourteenth. Sweetie and I decided to not fight the five to seven PM Baltimore traffic. Instead we got a good night's sleep at our hotel and left the next morning at three thirty AM, Central Daylight time (9/15/01, our fiftieth wedding anniversary). At least we were close together all day for our celebration, in our small Honda Civic.

Sweetie slept-walked to the car that morning and slept for the next three hours while I drove. She then took over the driving while I rested, and then I drove the rest of the way home. When we arrived at South Chicago at five thirty PM, we noticed the Saturday traffic to be lighter than on weekdays and decided to drive straight through the remaining four hours. We were able to sleep in our own bed that night. We covered 932 miles that day with only three stops for food and gas.

Meanwhile, on September seventeenth, we were informed by telephone from Attorney Godard's office, that we had achieved a defense verdict with the jurors finding Dr. Esposito not negligent in his care of Ms. Kinner. Two to three days later we received the letters reproduced below from Dr. Esposito and Attorney Godard. With that news, after all that happened in the previous week, I was able to take a deep breath. At least something went right during that time.

Drs. Esposito, Mayer, Hogan & Associates
Columbia, Maryland 21044

September 19, 2001
Dear Herbert,
This is a quick note of my appreciation. Having taken the time to review cases for quality assurance within the hospital and for local insurance companies, I have some appreciation of the amount of time it takes to diligently review charts and render an opinion. Dealing with plaintiff's attorneys by no means is a rewarding and enriching experience, and I certainly have a much greater appreciation and level of indebtedness to those who are willing to give of their time to help defend cases.
Sincerely, Mark Esposito, MD

Godard, West Adelman, Sheff & Smith LLC
Rockville, Maryland 20850

September 19, 2001
Re: Kinner v Esposito
Dear Dr. Sandmire
As you were advised by telephone by my office, the jury deliberated only for about forty-five minutes before returning their verdict on behalf of Dr. Esposito. The verdict form simply indicated that they found him "not negligent."
Obviously, your testimony was a key factor in our victory and both Dr. Esposito and I are extremely appreciative of your testimony, and all of the efforts that you put forth to assist in this defense.
I think that this verdict proves that we indeed reached a completely new era in the analysis and defense of shoulder dystocia cases.
Again, my sincere thanks and appreciation and I shall look forward to future opportunities to work with you.
Very truly yours, Gary A. Godard

CHAPTER 45

UWGB Chancellor's Award

OUR CONTRIBUTIONS TO the UWGB were recognized by University Chancellor Bruce Shepard, who on May 13, 2006 presented Crystal and me with the UWGB Chancellor's Award at the University's graduation ceremony. Along with the beautiful plaque was a printed recitation of the reasons we were selected:

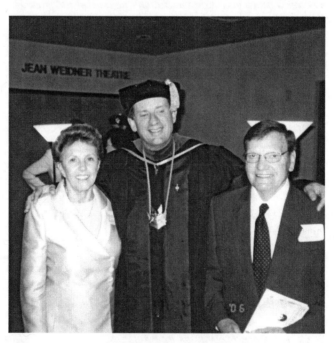

With Chancellor Bruce Shepard following Crystal and me jointly receiving the 2006 Chancellor's Award.

The Chancellor's Award
University of Wisconsin – Green Bay
Spring Commencement – May 13, 2006
HERBERT AND CRYSTAL SANDMIRE
Citation

Herbert and Crystal Sandmire illustrate the tremendous, positive force that engaged citizens can be for a developing university. The Sandmires were here at the beginning. Ever since. And even before. Let me explain.

Dr. Herbert Sandmire very likely had his former students among our first UWGB graduating class. For two decades, beginning in the late 1960s, Dr. Sandmire was a common lecturer in human biology.

That, nearly four decades later, a maturing UW-Green Bay counts pre-med, the natural sciences, and human biology among its very strong offerings, is in no small measure a reflection of the Sandmire family's help along the way.

They contributed: as early advisors and counselors.... by providing for student scholarships and gifts to the Founders Association.... and helping and housing medical students in residence here.

As private donors to this institution, they are all but without equal. Again, let me explain.

Today, the margin of excellence at UWGB is annually supported by the gifts of over 2,500 philanthropically inclined donors. On that list of thousands, Herb and Crystal's record for consistent giving is exceeded by only one individual, Chancellor Emeritus Ed Weidner, and, then by only one year.

The Sandmires' commitment to building UW-Green Bay extends beyond the health sciences... and to virtually every corner of the campus:

The Varsity Club and Phoenix Fund...
the Weidner Center construction....
the first capital campaign for student housing...
and more recently, Phuture Phoenix and the Student Events Center.

Crystal is a UWGB graduate, in Communications and the Arts. She is a charter member of the Founders, and a former officer.

I will also mention that their contributions to the larger community – its institutions and organizations – are similarly lengthy and impressive.

*Their combined list of awards and honors, to this point, was high-
lighted with Herb's selection, last May, as the recipient of the Ralph
Hawley Distinguished Service Award from the UW School of Medicine.*

*His outstanding contributions to his community, and profession
also include:*

---

41 scientific publications

---

*A dozen prestigious awards, several in recognition of his contri-
butions to the disciplines of gynecology and obstetrics, and nearly 50
years of courageous service in providing citizens of Northeast Wisconsin access to a full range of the best-available healthcare.*

*Our students, this university, indeed this entire community, owe
you a tremendous debt of gratitude. We acknowledge that debt today
and present to you, Herbert and Crystal Sandmire, the Chancellor's
Award of your University of Wisconsin – Green Bay.*

Signed, Bruce Shepard, Chancellor

CHAPTER 46

Charitable contributions

CRYSTAL AND I have always had a charitable giving philosophy. It is our opinion that our survival in this troubled world requires the presence of top-notch educational institutions; therefore, they are our number one priority for philanthropic giving. We annually donate to our named scholarships at St. Norbert College and the University of Wisconsin-Green Bay (UWGB). In addition we have several times made substantial gifts to the University of Wisconsin School of Medicine and Public Health.

Our second daughter, Yvonne, received a full gymnastics scholarship from Arizona State University (Title nine came just in time – hey, that rhymes). She subsequently became head women's gymnastics coach at Boise State University, serving there for 20 years prior to her retirement two years ago. We have shown our appreciation to both Arizona State and Boise State for the positive role they played in Yvonne's life by our annual contributions and by a Boise State scholarship in Yvonne's name.

In addition, we annually donate to Scholarships Incorporated, an organization that aids needy high school students in pursuing their college education. Crystal has also contributed to this organization by serving as its president in 1982 and on its selection committee for several years. The United Way and other organizations receive considerable annual donations as well.

CHAPTER 47

The long road to Paris

DURING THE COURSE of 2006, Dr. Claude Racinet, of Grenoble, France, began to correspond with me regarding our shared interest in shoulder dystocia (SD) and brachial plexus injury (BPI). He had read some of my publications and was an enthusiastic supporter of my ideas on BPI causation.

In a December 3, 2006 email, Dr. Racinet stated, "if you can speak French (even slowly) we could invite you to describe the medico-legal problems associated with brachial plexus palsy (BPP) and the answers to give at the court." The entire email follows:

> Dear Dr. Sandmire,
> I apologize for my poor english but I hope you are able to understand my message. I would first thank you for sending all your papers about SD and BPP.
> The National College (french) of obstetricians and gynecologists (CNGOF) has decided on my recommendations to organize a session for medical experts in GO in December 2007 in Paris. We would want you to give updated information about the main problems encountered in law courts. If you can speak in french (even slowly), we could invite you to describe the medico-legal problems associated with BPP and the answers to give at the court. But we first need to know the amount of your fees and conditions. If it is not possible, is there anybody in your medical team who is able to speak french and to express your recommendations?
> I'm reading your papers and will write later to you to give my opinion. Thank you for answering on the eventual possibility to respond to the invitation of the CNGOF.
> Sincerely yours, Claude Racinet

Meanwhile, I continued to share my opinions on BPI causation as illustrated by the following email:

> Dear Dr. Racinet,
> When shoulder dystocia (SD) is present, 80% of all brachial plexus injuries affect the anterior arm. When the posterior arm is injured it indicates **transient** obstruction of the posterior shoulder as the baby travels down the birth canal. We know that the posterior shoulder can no longer be obstructed by the promontory of the sacrum (after the head is out of the birth canal) because the neck cannot be stretched that far. The distance from the promontory to the pelvic outlet is 11 to 12 cms. Interestingly, when there is an injury to the posterior arm there is no associated SD in 67% of those injuries (Gherman).
> We described the mechanism for the posterior arm injury in our 2002 article entitled "Erb's palsy without shoulder dystocia." I will send it to you, by regular mail, at Marie-Ange Mernet's address, as well as all of our articles relating to SD. In addition, I will include plaintiffs' expert memos 11 – 17 which I have authored to help attorneys who are defending physicians. These, without some of the articles referred to, will also be sent to you by email. Also I will send some power point screens which we have used as exhibits at legal trials.
> I have recently sent you by regular mail, an article by Stirrat together with some questions (also sent Pl. Exp. Memo 17 authored by myself – do you agree with my views?). I eagerly look forward to your response.
> Sincerely, Herbert F. Sandmire MD

Dr. Racinet sent an email on February 5, 2007, indicating the Board of CNGOF was considering his recommendation to have me speak at their annual meeting in December of 2007:

> Dear Dr. Sandmire,
> First, I apologize for not responding immediately after your precedent email. Your questions are so complex that I need a period of reflexion. But your explanations for the pathogenesis of spontaneous BP are very attractive.... I asked the Board of CNGOF for inviting you in Paris. The response is on study: It seems that this would be possible but it depends of the cost of the travel from your residence to Paris. Do you have an idea about the cost?

Thank you for mailing all your papers and others, particularly the plaintiff's expert memos. I'll write to you before the end of February, but I'm waiting for the estimated cost of your trip.
Sincerely yours, Claude Racinet

In the meantime I notified him and the executive board of CNGOF that I would be unable to deliver my lecture in the French language:

Dear Dr. Racinet,
I have had second thoughts regarding addressing the French College of Obstetrics and Gynecology in the French language. I believe the only way that would happen is to have an interpreter. I notify you at this time in order that, if you choose, you can seek another speaker.
Sincerely, Herbert F. Sandmire MD

The board of CNGOF decreed that all speakers at the meeting must deliver their lectures in the French language:

Dear Herbert Sandmire,
The board of CNGOF has decided that all the speakers at the Meeting on Medico-legal aspects in Obstetrics, devoted exclusively to french experts, should imperatively speak in french. Unfortunately, as you told me you could not speak in french, we will not have the opportunity for you to meet us in Paris, and an expert from Paris (aware of your papers) will talk on the topic.
I was very delighted to exchange some emails with you and I send you a paper in french where I am trying to synthesize the current pathogenesis, revisited by H Sandmire, about BPP. I'll hope we continue to exchange further by mail.
Best regards, CR

We continued exchanging our views on BPI causation. In addition, Claude informed me of the research of Domenico Pecorari, M.D., the leading authority in Italy regarding BPI causation. I began to work through my own concepts of BPI causation, reducing them to writing, and then passing them on to Racinet, Pecorari and three authorities in the United States, Hankins, Gherman and Morrison, to get their opinions. They all agreed with the logic of my views, and therefore I added each of their names as supporting co-authors of my paper: "Newborn brachial plexus injuries: the twisting and extension of the fetal head as contributing causes."

Our paper was accepted for publication in the *Journal of Obstetrics and Gynecology* in 2008, with an editorial comment that "Perhaps the most important recent paper is that of Sandmire et al. (2008)." In the meantime, I had two more BPI papers published: "Newborn brachial plexus palsy" and "Controversies surrounding the causes of brachial plexus injury." The latter article was translated into Italian and also published in the June/July 2009 issue of the *Giornaali Italiano di Oestricia Ginecologia*, an exceedingly uncommon event.

Surprisingly, Claude Racinet sent me a January 31, 2010 email reissuing the invitation for me to now present two lectures at the CNGOF annual meeting in December 2010 in Paris, both to be delivered in English:

> *Dear Herbert,*
>
> *I just obtained to-day by phone the CNGOF's agreement for your invitation to the 34emes Journees nationales du CNGOF from 8 to 11 December 2010 at Paris (CNGOF: College National des Gynecologues-Obstetriciens Francais).*
>
> *The conditions are the following:*
>
> 1. *For your trip: you will have the choice between purchasing yourself your ticket from Green Bay to Paris (via Chicago?) in economic class (return on Sunday is less expensive), or putting the travel agency of CNGOF (Colloquium) in charge of doing the reservation?*
>
> 2. *Your hotel reservation for 4 nights (from Tuesday 7 to Friday 10) will be booked on behalf of Colloquium, but if you have the opportunity to stay more you could manage that directly with the hotel or better through Colloquiuim...*
>
> 3. *You will have to give 2 lectures within the context of a Journey-Thursday 9/12 – devoted to medico-legal problems. First, the obstetrician audience is interested by your extensive experience in the court of laws and will receive with great interest your responses to the main controversies in the field of BPI (45 min, including 10 minutes for questions). Second, we are also interested in the ACOG's Grievance Committee, which we may want to duplicate in CNGOF! We need to have a short description of how it functions and a report of some cases (warning, censure and professional and legal consequences for the "expert" who testifies in violation professional recommendations). 45 min. including 15 min. for discussion.*
>
> *Do you agree with these conditions?*
>
> *Sincerely yours, Claude*

Sweetie began immediately checking flight times and costs (was she excited or not?) and emailed all of the females in our family, inviting them to accompany us on our road to Paris:

> *Dear Daughters- in-law and Daughters,*
> *We have emailed to you the letter we got from Claude Racinet saying the trip is on for Herb to speak to their National Medical Organization (CNGOF). We will have more information in a few weeks according to this letter. In the meantime (so you can be thinking about plans), you are invited to go with us (Herb and six women). We will work out details, but we are thinking we will pay your airfare over and back and your rooms while we are there. Your excursions, shopping, incidentals and meals are on your own.*
> *The meeting is from Wed. through Sat., December seven to ten. Herb will be speaking on Thurs. Since he does not understand French, he probably would not attend any other days. We may go a couple days early (before he speaks). Anyway, at this time, we are thinking the trip would be seven days. Perhaps each of you can be looking into airline possibilities. Tentatively, we checked air possibilities from here with United (thru Chicago), economy class, is just under $1000 – leaves here at 2:35 pm, getting to Chicago at 3:32pm, leaving Chicago at 6:28 and getting to Paris at 9:40am the next morning. Evidently it is non-stop from Chicago.*
> *That's about it for now. We will keep you updated as we get more information.*
> *Love, H & C – Mom and Dad S.*

Later on, when the men in our family got wind of the Paris excursion, led primarily by son-in-law Cary, they began clamoring for a similar all-expense-paid trip. I offered them a weekend bowling trip to Seymour or Pulaski (their choice), hopefully to be scheduled with the annual cow chip toss in those cities.

Initially, the invitee list to Paris included Sweetie, Cheryl, Yvonne, Lisa, Karen and Beth. Later in that year, 2010, while having dinner at the Green Bay Country Club, Kevin said "what about Crystie [our granddaughter], isn't she a female?" I said, "That's right." Neither of us had thought beyond daughters and daughter-in-laws but promptly extended the invitation to Crystie to join us, with the approval of her parents, of course.

Daughter-in-law Lisa had to forego the trip in order to give support to her sister, recently diagnosed with breast cancer.

Our flight to Paris on December 5th via Minneapolis went well. Our time in Paris continued through December 12th. We had nothing scheduled for our first day except checking in to our charming Hotel Cecelia and resting after a long, overnight flight.

The next day we had a half-day city tour in a van for just our family with a great driver and guide, Fred. He did a super job showing us the highlights of Paris so that we could go back later to spend more time in places of special interest. That afternoon, Sweetie and I traveled by train to CNIT, the sight of the meeting, to review my power point screens with Dr. Racinet, who was to give a limited amount of translation during the presentation of my two lectures. Because of a technology glitch, we had to return the next day. At lunchtime of that day, Sweetie and I were invited to have lunch with the president of CNGOF and some other officers of the organization.

My two lectures were presented on Thursday, December 9th: 1) "Controversies surrounding brachial plexus injury causation," and 2) "The functioning of the ACOG Grievance Committee." Both lectures seemed to be well-received, with my English language delivered in a slow, understandable fashion as revealed by the nodding of heads as I made my main points. That same evening all of my family members were invited to a Gala at the Eiffel Tower for a gourmet dinner and to witness my induction as a member in honor into le College National des Gynecologists et Obstetrics Francois. Some of the members of our family said it was a "magical evening".

One might ask, *"What did Dr. Sandmire have to offer that could not have been presented by a French obstetrician?"* I surmise that it related to my multiple publications outlining the indirect evidence for the maternal labor forces as the likely cause of BPI and my extensive legal experience. The indirect evidence was significantly important, as there was no possibility of designing an ethical study that could determine or refute that BPI was caused by excessive, clinician-applied traction – a claim that had been made repeatedly from the early 1900s until the 1970s despite there being no direct or indirect evidence for that as the cause.

The first article leading to my suspicion that maternal labor forces were the cause of BPI was Gordon's 1973 article reporting that 49 percent of newborns with permanent BPI (PBPI) were the product of normal vaginal deliveries that were not complicated by shoulder dystocia (SD). If physician-applied traction were the cause, how could one explain why 49 percent of newborns with PBPI were from normal, non-traction deliveries?

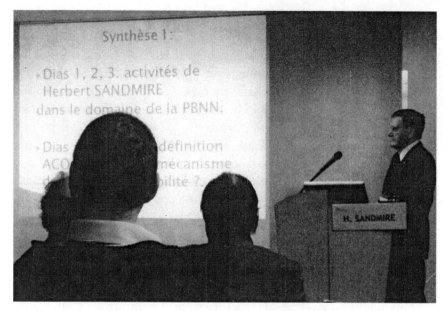

Lecturing to the members of Le College National des Gynecologists et Obstetricians Francais. (December 9, 2010)

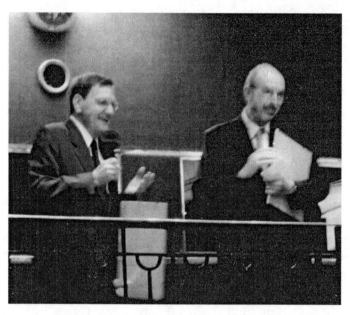

Induction as a member in honor into Le College National des Gynecologist et Obstetricians Francais at an Eiffel Tower Gala. (December 9, 2010)

Gordon's findings were confirmed by my own research and by that of 20 other authors during the ensuing 25 years. Other significant indirect evidence that maternal labor forces cause PBPI include a four-fold increase in PBPI in cases when the second pushing stage of labor was more rapid than normal, the existence of the same incidence of PBPI between highly experienced and less experienced physicians, the unchanging frequency of PBPI over the past 80 years despite the common admonition to be gentle in our delivery technique, the equal frequencies (1:1200) of PBPI in Canada (where strong downward traction was used in 37 percent of their deliveries complicated by SD) and the United States (where SD was overcome with conventional maneuvers and no excessive traction), and the observation that 32-39 percent of PBPI involved the posterior (back side of the) arm during the delivery process, which, because of the distance from the posterior pelvic inlet to the vaginal outlet, can only be caused by transient obstruction before the fetal head begins to exit the birth canal. Finally, despite training for the management of SD with birth simulation and a rising cesarean rate, the incidence of PBPI had remained unchanged over a ten-year period. Each of these indirect pieces of evidence can be seen as individual parts of the puzzle which, when assembled together, strongly suggest that the cause of PBPI is the maternal labor forces.

Amazingly, Dr. Racinet had reviewed all of my papers on this subject, also available on Pub Med, and Google. Pub Med is able to provide the titles of all of my and other physicians' publications. The world is indeed shrinking.

Coming home:

On Sunday, December 12th, we went to the Paris airport by taxi only to find out that our flight had been cancelled due to weather conditions in Minneapolis. We then booked a flight to Detroit and on to Green Bay. We sat in the Green Bay-bound plane in Detroit for three hours waiting for the wind to decrease. It didn't, and that flight was also cancelled.

We then were told that, because of the backlog, it would be two days before a flight to Green Bay would be available. After waiting for one and one-half hours in the taxi line, we headed to the Embassy Suites hotel in Livonia, Michigan, 35 miles from Detroit. This was the closest available room we could find.

Two days later, we arrived home following an uneventful flight. In an attempt to avoid being frustrated, I made my usual comment, "You have to be alive somewhere on this earth – so what is so bad about Livonia, Michigan in a nice Embassy Suites hotel."

The younger members of our family had many warm memories of Paris.

Paris Memories

Beth's memories: *In 1992, I had my first experience visiting Paris with my husband and son. Granted, Alec was only 6 months in the womb, but he came along nonetheless. Dave and I were backpacking through Europe and we had only 36 hours to take in the city. So, when I found out in 2010 that my in-laws were gifting a WHOLE week's trip to Paris with all the girls in the family, I was thrilled!*

Herb and Sweetie treated the girls to a beautiful stay in the most "chic" city in the world. Our Hotel Cecilia was charming. It was located in a wonderful position near all the areas we wanted to visit. The Metro station was only a block away, which made the whole city accessible to us.

We had a couple of days to be tourists and visit the classic sites at a relaxing pace (e.g. Montemarte, Notre Dame, Champs Elysees, and Le Arc de Triomphe). We toured during the day and caught up with each other's families over a bottle of wine and cheese and crackers at night in our hotel room. The fourth day of our trip, we got to see Herb and Crystal in their element (one does not function without the other, in my opinion). Herb presented lectures at the College National des Gynecologists et Obstetricians, Francais (the French version of the American College of Obstetricians and Gynecologists). I thought it was a wonderful moment for my daughter to see her grandfather and grandmother doing what they do best, teaching others and being exceptional role models as people who change the world for the better. Then, in the evening, the Gala at le Eiffel Tower occurred. Again, it was an important reminder to me and my daughter that hard work has its rewards. Crystie had her first sip of champagne while in the company of her family, seeing her grandfather accepted as a "member in honor" into the College National des Gynecologists et Obstetricians, Francais and the added benefit of viewing Paris from the Eiffel Tower.

The whole experience will not be forgotten. Beautiful sites, great food and a loving family: priceless.

Cheryl's memories: *Paris is one of the most beautiful large cities I have ever visited. It is also one of the largest cities that I have visited and actually seems much smaller. This is for two reasons. The first being that Paris is made up of lots of small neighborhoods, so you always feel you are in a smaller place. I love the individual neighborhoods, each with its own characteristics and sights to see. Montmarte was especially nice. It is where many of the past and present artists live, work and hang out. Being an artist myself, this part of town really resonated with me. It is very quaint, with its tiny shops, markets and cafes, and the artists paint outside, right on the tiny picturesque square.*

The second reason Paris seems much smaller than it is, is the fabulous underground transportation system they have. For two Euros and 15 minutes of your time, you can travel from one part of the city to another without ever having to get in your car. Very impressive and a super "green" way to get from place to place. When is our country going to catch on to mass transportation??

My final impression of beautiful Paris is that it has so many inspirational works of art that it is impossible to walk around town without being thoroughly impressed, amazed and enchanted by it.

I loved every minute I was there.

Thank you Mom and Dad for making it possible!

Crystie's memories: *Dear Grandma and Grandpa the Great,*

First of all, Congratulations on your award! It was great to be there with you guys when you accepted it! I loved the whole trip and being with the girls in the family. One of my favorite things we did was eating dinner at the Eiffel Tower. That was a great dinner. And I liked the bus tour, except for the part when Cher lost her bag – good thing she found it. Thank you so much for inviting me and my Mom.

Love, Crystie

Karen's memories: *Over the years, Herb and Crystal have treated Kevin and me to vacations all over the globe, from the Mediterranean to Hawaii, Alaska to the Panama Canal. I have enjoyed them all, but among my favorites was our most recent trip together to France. From the moment they extended the invitation, I looked forward with excitement to a week-long adventure in Paris.*

It was fun to start the morning with the seven of us, sharing our plans for the day while drinking cafe au lait and eating chocolate croissants (my favorite). It was a real pleasure to be able to spend time with the women of our family while leisurely exploring the city by day as a group, or at times on our own. The evenings at the Hotel Cecelia, back again with Herb and Sweetie, were delightfully relaxing as we enjoyed a glass of wine while recounting the highlights of our day.

I have so many wonderful memories of our time in Paris, yet there are several that come to mind before others. I was overwhelmed by the history, architecture and art of the city. Of the museums and galleries that we toured, the Musee D'Orsey was my favorite. At Notre Dame, I felt as if I were stepping back in time, imagining not only the masons who designed and built the cathedral but also the people who had entered its vast interior over the ages. I loved the rainy evening we spent ambling through St. Germaine, picking our way over the narrow cobblestone streets, peering into tiny shops and stopping for a bite to eat at one of the many quaint patisseries. Walking along the Champs de l'Elysee at night, the wet pavement reflecting the blue lights hanging from the chestnut trees that lined the boulevard was truly enchanting.

Despite the language barrier and the differences in medical practices in Europe and the U.S., when we attended the OB/GYN conference, it was inspirational to watch and listen as both groups of physicians shared their knowledge and opinions about the topic at hand. The grand finale of the trip was the gourmet dinner held in the Eiffel Tower, overlooking the Champs de l'Elysee as it sparkled under the evening lights, while we drank French champagne; it was a surreal experience. Watching Herb as he was inducted as a member of honor into Le College National des Gynecologists et Obstetricians Francais was a proud moment and the perfect ending to an unforgettable trip.

Vonnie's memories : *In keeping with their tradition of giving their kids incredible experiences, my generous parents decided to invite all of the women in our family to Paris!*

The chance to experience such a beautiful, historic city with close family would have been enough, but it was even more special being able to witness my Dad's presentation to and honor by the Society of French Obstetricians & Gynecologists. At the presentation, I learned that my father is considered the world's leading authority on shoulder dystocia/brachial plexus injury (a condition that can cause partial paralysis) in newborn babies. Dr. Claude Racinet told me that Dad's research & presentation "will positively change the way medicine is practiced in France."

The highlight of our trip was the gala in the restaurant at the Eiffel Tour. The gourmet food, incredible view, interesting conversations and inspiring ceremony honoring Dad & other physicians whose work had improved medical practice was almost surreal. I couldn't believe we were in such a beautiful, historic place, witnessing such an important event. I have always been proud of my parents (and anyone who knows them understands that Dad's research is always a cooperative effort with my Mom), but this was the icing on the cake!

I will always remember this very special trip. We were able to visit the Louvre, L'Arc de Triumph, the palace at Versailles (including the Hall of Mirrors where the World War II peace treaty was signed), Champs d'Elysees and other famous Paris sites. Together, we enjoyed breakfasts and happy hours at Hotel Cecilia and dinners out at small cafes. We learned a little French and figured out the Metro and train systems. And we experienced the biggest snowfall Paris had seen in 20 years. I will be eternally grateful for this wonderful opportunity to share such a special place and time with my family.

Dian Page memorialized our trip to Paris in the following article:

Sandmire honored at Eiffel Tower fete
Dian Page of Green Bay Press Gazette, 1-25-2011

At a gala dinner on the first floor of the Eiffel Tower in Paris, Dr. Herbert Sandmire of Green Bay was recently inducted as a member in honor into Le College National des Gynecologists et Obstetricians Francais, the French version of American College of Obstetricians and Gynecologists.

Sandmire's contributions as a practicing physician, academic professor and legal expert were cited during his induction ceremony also attended by his wife, Crystal Sandmire; daughters, Cheryl Sandmire and Yvonne Sandmire Hattabaugh; daughters-in-law, Karen Sandmire and Beth Sandmire and granddaughter, Crystie Sandmire.

The event followed Sandmire's two lectures at the annual meeting of the French National College of Gynecologists and Obstetricians. His lecture titles were "Controversies Surrounding Brachial Plexus Injury (BPI) Causation" and the "Functioning of the American College of Obstetricians and Gynecologists Grievance Committee," which the French may duplicate.

According to the doctor, the brachial plexus is the network of nerves located in the neck that supply the muscles controlling movements of the arm and shoulder. When injured during the normal birth process, the affected muscle is paralyzed.

He was introduced by French obstetrician Dr. Claude Racinet from Grenoble, who called him "the world's leading authority on BPI causation because he deduced the correct cause of BPI from seven separate pieces of indirect evidence. The findings presented by Herb will

275

definitely impact the practice of medicine in our country."

Following 51 years in Green Bay, Sandmire retired from his practice at Ob-gyn Associates of Green Bay in May 2010.

The finale

July 8, 2010
Dear Dr. Sandmire,
I want to thank you for being my doctor for over __50__ years !!! You were always there to help me. I wish you the best in your retirement.
Mary Neville
P.S. __You are the greatest__ !!!

CPSIA information can be obtained at www.ICGtesting.com
Printed in the USA
LVOW071908280512

283632LV00002B/2/P